ease into fitness

ease into fitness

DIANA MORAN

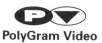

PolyGram Video

BOXTREE

First published in the UK in 1993 by
Boxtree Limited
Broadwall House
21 Broadwall
London SE1 9PL

13579108642

Text © copyright Diana Moran, 1993.
Photographs © copyright Rick Wilson,
except photos on p.10 and p.64 © copyright Peter Cranham,
and photo on p.124-, property of Poole Hospital NHS Trust.

Designed and typeset by Blackjacks, London

Printed and bound in Great Britain by
Butler & Tanner Limited, Frome

Cover photograph courtesy of Polygram Video.
Leotard and tights supplied by Carita of Denmark.
Phone or send for a free catalogue to Carita House of Stapeley, Nantwich,
Cheshire. Telephone: 0270 627722.

CONTENTS

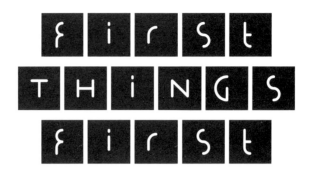

itness and health are not the same thing. Although someone may look fit, and think they are fit, closer examination and some specific 'fitness tests' could well prove otherwise. It may simply be a matter of failing to meet the target in, say, a cardiovascular test for someone of their sex and age or perhaps a deeper underlying health problem may be revealed. Things aren't always as they first seem and appearances can be deceptive.

Total fitness is made up of five basic components: nutritional fitness, medical fitness, mental fitness, emotional and social fitness.

A totally fit person possessing all these components will have no problems in meeting the demands life make, and will still have reserves to draw upon in an emergency.

The exercise section of this book concentrates on one of these components, physical fitness. This is itself divided into five components.

The first component is **cardiovascular fitness**. This is what gives us stamina. It governs the efficiency of our heart and lungs. We can improve our cardiovascular capacity by means of the Aerobic section of our exercise programme when we make our bodies work hard between 60 to 80 per cent of our estimated maximum heart rate. This 'training zone' can be calculated and adjusted to suit individual needs.

Muscular strength is the second component and is the ability of a muscle to exert maximum force to overcome a resistance. This can be improved by gradually increasing the resistance in an exercise by using alternative positions or

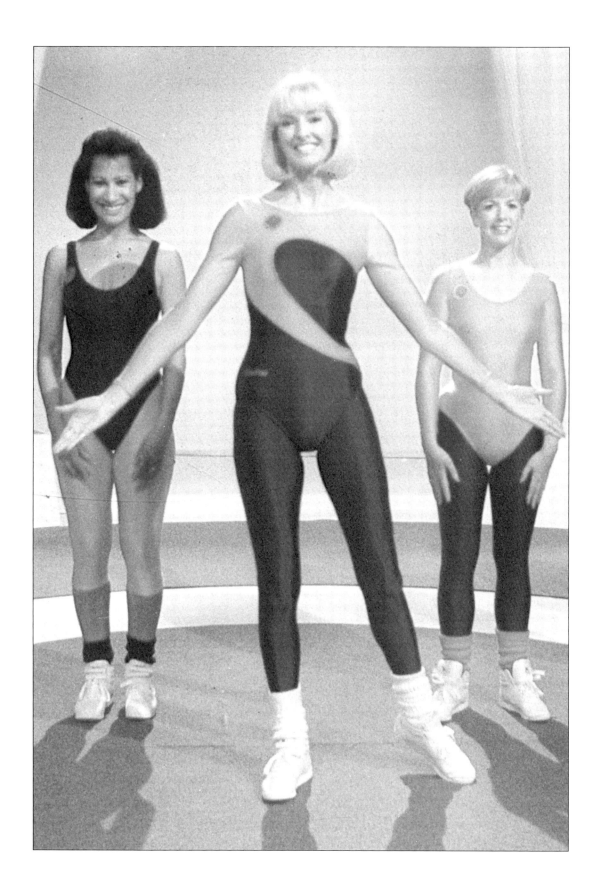

weights according to individual requirements. It is developed in the M.S.E (Muscular Strength and Endurance) section of our work-out.

Muscular endurance, the third component, is also enhanced by the exercises given in the M.S.E section. It concerns the ability of a muscle (or groups of muscles) to exert force to overcome a resistance for an extended period of time. How long and how many times we do an exercise will increase our muscular endurance.

The fourth component, **flexibility**, enables us to put our muscles and joints through their full range of movements with ease. We encourage this in the warm up, Short Stretches and in the Relax/Stretch sections, working the muscles more intensively to enhance their flexibility still further. A typical example of this would be the work we do on our hamstrings.

The final component of physical fitness is **motor fitness**. This concerns our skill and ability in controlling movement, balance, speed, co-ordination, agility, and capacity to react quickly. Our motor fitness is improved through all sections of our work-out, but particularly during the Warm Up and Aerobic sections.

But, remember: we should all aim for total fitness rather than just physical fitness. I hope that this book will put you on the right road to achieving this. We can all improve our physical fitness to some degree by exercise but there are other factors which will play an important part in achieving overall fitness.

What we eat and whether we smoke are important factors, as are age and sex. The medical history of our parents and family may also affect our own ability to achieve total fitness.

There are also three main body types. None of us is an exact 'type', but I am sure you'll recognise yourself as a variation on the theme of one of these:

Ectomorphs are usually tall and slender with slim bones, narrow shoulders and hips, and not much fat or muscle.

Endomorphs tend to be shorter and more rounded, with wide hips and larger bones.

Mesomorphs can be tall or short and have a more triangular, athletic shape with broad, well-developed shoulders, narrow waists and strong hips.

No matter how hard we diet and exercise, which may improve our physical appearance, our basic body type remains unchanged.

We are, of course, all unique and as we progress, results will differ from one person to another. For this reason alone it's important not to set your goals too high and aim for the impossible. You'll only end up disappointed and forever chasing a dream. Know your limits and success is sure to come.

Good luck!

WHAT IS FITNESS?

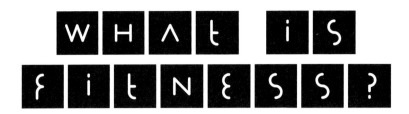

As a young girl and a teenager, I was as fit as fit could be. My West Country childhood was packed full of healthy exercise. Show me an ice-rink and I'd be on it. Show me a swimming pool and I'd plough up and down till the cows came home! I was no slouch on the athletics track either and, all modesty aside, I played a mean game of tennis. I didn't realise how lucky I was.

Then at the age of 20 I got married. Within a handful of years I had two beautiful baby boys to look after. All that fresh air and fun had been replaced by nappy pails and pram-pushing. But, my goodness, it was still exercise. And it still kept me fit. Anyone who's chased after a couple of active toddlers will know precisely what I mean! If, and

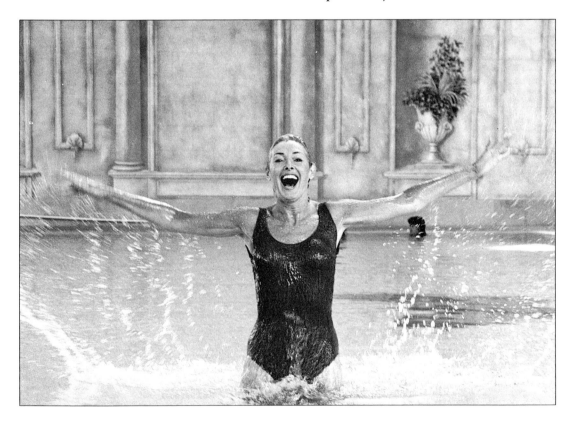

when, they gave up the struggle, I'd go straight out into the garden that I loved and put some honest toil into the flowers, fruit and vegetables. That, too, kept me fit.

At the age of 29, I learnt one of life's simplest lessons: you can't take your health and fitness for granted. I was in hospital recovering from an operation, and when I looked at myself in the mirror I realised I wasn't the person I used to be. With the best of intentions I'd fallen into the trap that beckons all young mums. I'd become the dust-bin that swallowed up all the boys' leftovers; I'd let them (and therefore me) eat junk food and chocolate; and I'd forgotten to look after myself.

To be honest, I didn't like what I saw. Don't forget, ten years previously I'd been at the peak of physical fitness. Now I saw a woman who looked overweight, slow and lethargic, and whose skin looked pale and dull. I don't get angry often, but here I was, just 29 years old, and all I could see was a woman well into middle age.

As soon as I left hospital, I set myself the task of finding my way back to the fitness I'd once enjoyed. But this was 25 years ago, and books on the subject were few and far between. I tried yoga, but my body wasn't supple enough. Then I found out about the Keep Fit Association and the League of Health and Beauty. I enjoyed learning the movements and exercises that were then in fashion. I also read every book or magazine article on health and fitness I could lay my hands on. Then I put the whole lot in a melting pot and came up with a set of exercises that would suit me and my busy life-style.

Just one year later I was in hospital again, this time with acute appendicitis. Exercise had nothing to do with this problem – but diet certainly did. The doctor who saw me through introduced me to yet another way of thinking about my own body. I'd understood about exercise, but now he was telling me about high-fibre diets and keeping regular. His words of advice fuelled a new interest in nutrition,

TOP TIP

You do enough for your family and friends already. Don't be the dust-bin that swallows up all the leftovers and samples all the cooking You'd be surprised how quickly the calories mount up.

TOP TIP

Eat vegetables raw and keep some prepared in the fridge to nibble crudite-style. If you're hooked on cooked vegetables, steam them, microwave them, or use a wok. But don't boil them away to nothing!

and once I'd left hospital I began my search for the recipe for a healthy diet.

After convalescing, I went back to my career as a model. All my friends noticed the difference in me. Exercise and careful eating had given me a new-found enthusiasm, a zest for life and a healthy glow. It didn't take long for my girl-friends to cotton on and start quizzing me for tips on keeping fit. My career as a keep fit lady had begun. Soon I found myself being invited to go public with my new-found knowledge. My first guinea-pigs were Butlin's holiday-makers at Minehead and Barry Island.

Over the following years I started to build up the routines and exercises that I'm now well known for. But I didn't make the mistake of slavishly following just one method. I picked and mixed from all over the place to find exercises that not only kept me in shape but made me feel good too. I also decided to walk more, swim, cycle, and tackle the garden with new gusto. Even when I was decorating or dancing, I realised that these too were natural forms of exercise.

On the food front I was learning to be a lot more sensible about my diet. I ate less fat and more fibre and lots more fresh fruit and vegetables. I cut down on red meats and chose chicken or fish instead. I continued to have a glass or two of white wine once in a while. and I never smoked. To be honest, I'd learnt to think of my body as the home I live in. And who in their right mind sets fire to their own home? Smokers do!

It was all common sense really and probably best summed up by a wonderfully fit eighty-year-old woman I met on my keep fit travels. when I asked her how she'd kept so trim and agile she said simply, "My dear Diana, if you don't use it, you might lose it!"

Being fit, as I am sure you'll soon agree, brings new quality and buzz to everyday life. When your body's fit, you can make it do what you want it to do for as long as you need.

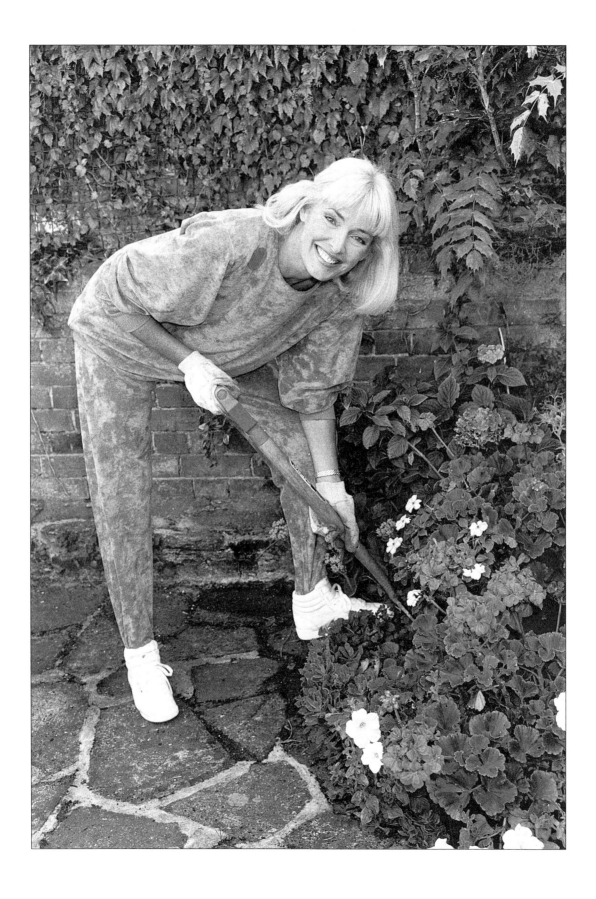

And during my 30s I really did need to be fit. Not only was I teaching others my way to fitness, but my modelling career had gone into overdrive – I was travelling the world doing one fashion shoot after another.

Now, a model's life really is hard work and it's certainly not as glamorous as it's cracked up to be. The locations can be idyllic but facilities non-existent. There's many a time I've had to change clothes behind a couple of bushes or crunched up on the back seat of a car!

One memorable occasion still sticks in my mind. We were doing a fashion show at Cheltenham's Pump Rooms – the changing room was actually the kitchen. On the catwalk everything looked sweetness and light. Backstage, as usual, it was complete mayhem with girls rushing in and out, arms and legs flailing, dressers primping and preening and 'You're on in 30 seconds!' At times like this, all modesty is cast to the winds.

Unfortunately on this occasion we sprang a leak – the kitchens that is, not the models! The plumbers were called in and went about their business while we girls continued dashing in and out pulling off one frock and hopping into another. None of the men uttered a word of complaint. But I did overhear one say to his mate, 'Cor, I thought my wife was quite normal until I saw this lot!' The backstage show we'd put on for him and his mates was indeed a treat. What he'd seen was a group of healthy happy girls at the peak of fitness looking just like nature intended.

Indeed nature did intend us to be lithe, strong and supple. And up till our grandparents' day, the hard slog of everyday life kept men and women much fitter than all too many of their grandchildren. Nowadays it's easy to use only our brains instead of our brawn.

Just think back a bit. A man's life was much more physi-cally demanding then. He probably walked to work, no cars then, and more often than not his occupation would be heavy manual labour. Exhausted at the end of the day, he'd

go home and sit down for a well-deserved rest. But not for
long. The garden or the allotment beckoned and animals
had to be fed.

Life was just as physically demanding for his wife at home,
with all the household chores of washing and scrubbing and
looking after the children. Don't forget there were no
labour-saving devices in those days, and certainly no television to slump down in front of after a hard day's work.

Of course the quality of our lives has improved in many
ways since our grandparents' days. Work tends to be far less
arduous and there's much more time for enjoyment. But all
too many people don't make proper use of that time and let
their bodies slip out of condition. Our bodies were designed
to work with innate rhythm and grace. Just watch a gardener
using the traditional method of scything through long grass
and you'll see what I mean. Compare that with working life
spent hunched up in front of a VDU screen or tied to an
assembly line. No wonder one of the curses of modern age
is the bad back.

There is a lot more to being fit and well than just not
being ill. It's a whole approach to life designed to reduce
the risk of serious illness. And when, as happened to me
a few years ago, you cannot avoid becoming ill, your body
is fitter and better equipped to fight and win your battle
for you.

But just how fit are we? Sadly, according to a recent
Gallup Poll, we in the West aren't very fit at all. In spite of
all the information and encouragement to exercise, only
half the male and a third of the female population do
between one and three hours' exercise a week. Things are
slightly better on the food front though and there are
encouraging signs that over the past five years the message
has got through to reduce the intake of fatty foods, red
meat, sugar and white bread.

Fortunately, too, statistics show a marked decrease in the
number of deaths from smoking. Lung cancer is less preva-

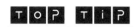

lent among women over 50, but proportionately more younger women than men are taking up cigarettes. Women may be strong in so many other areas but once they're hooked they find it even harder than men to kick the habit.

My own childhood was devastated by the early death of my mother from a stroke. She was only in her 40s and had smoked heavily. Forty years ago, though, the dangers of smoking weren't recognised. But I still wonder whether her death and the agony of bereavement could have been prevented. Today there can be no excuse. The message is loud and clear: smoking kills. Yet one in ten young girls still smoke. What of the future for them? And what avoidable tragedies lie ahead?

The sad fact of life is that in spite of the limited amount of exercise that's enjoyed by less than half of the adult population, and the slow improvements in the nations nutritional habits, we in Britain are still among the unhealthiest people in the Western World. We can only hope that more and more people learn to exercise regularly and take care about what they eat. Together with the increase in mass-screening and cancer prevention programmes, thousands of lives could and should be saved by these simple measures.

And early death is always a tragedy. A hundred years ago, if someone 'died young' he or she might have been in their 30s or 40s. Today we mean in the 50s or 60s. In the future we can hope still to be active and healthy in our 70s and 80s.

Of course we can't stop the inevitable. We will all have to die at some time and some of us will literally wear out sooner than others. But modern medicine has removed the threat of so many of the diseases that plagued previous generations. Antibiotics and vaccines have all but put paid to the devastating effects of diseases that were the major killers little more than 50 years ago – TB, influenza, whooping cough, diphtheria, scarlet fever and measles. Interestingly, the diseases that kill today such as cancer and heart disease didn't even appear in statistics until the 30s.

Statistics can, of course, be misleading. Take for instance the figures for breast cancer. One in ten women will be affected by breast cancer and subsequently die from it and despite screening programmes and public awareness the figures appear to be rising. The reason for that though is simple. We're living longer and many women are reaching their 40s, 50s and 60s, the ages when breast cancer is most likely to present itself.

So, barring accidents and genetic inheritance, we should all live longer. Exercise and diet will not necessarily increase our life-span, but they will certainly increase the quality of our lives. If you went into a shop and bought a machine, you'd expect it to work as the maker intended it. Our bodies are infinitely more complex than any machine. But with a little care and effort we can maintain them just as their maker intended.

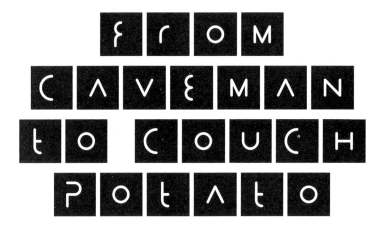

FROM CAVEMAN TO COUCH POTATO

3 ack in the mists of time, our cave-dwelling ancestors had to be fit to survive. Yesterday's Rambo had to stalk and kill his own food and be ever ready to do battle with his enemies. A strong lithe body and a pair of fast heels were his chief requirements.

Over the years, our Rambo got beyond the grunting stage. His body was still a finely tuned instrument and his mind as alert as ever, but he learnt to harness animals and enlist their help in daily back-breaking work.

In his own way, he'd discovered leisure time. But what did he do with it? Most of the time he perfected the skills that were essential to his survival, like hunting and archery. He also discovered his own voice and began to use communication rather than a club to attract a mate.

As he evolved, many of his previous pursuits took a ritual significance. Dance and competitive shows of strength and endurance were symbols of excellence and honour.

Just how important these early pursuits of physical excellence were to our predecessors is magnificently demonstrated in the founding of the original Olympic Games. Countries which otherwise might have been at war settled their differences on field and track. Laurel wreaths were more prized than a bloody sword.

Many of the games we play and enjoy today hark back to those early beginnings, like running, swimming, wrestling and equestrian sports.

The ritual dance survived through pagan times and, modified over the years, became the folk dances that distinguish every nation. In our part of the world, the Scots and the Irish are justly proud of their traditional dances and the English can look to their Morris Men and Mummers as fine examples of a centuries-old tradition that has survived and continues to flourish in the twentieth century.

Even the British Navy is still dancing. On high days and holidays they perform the traditional hornpipe. Now, it's a wonderful piece of entertainment. A century ago it was a brilliant way of keeping a crew fit as they sailed the seven seas. You might even say that they should be credited with the invention of aerobic dancing! Nowadays, by the way, the Services are into keeping fit in a big way and I and my fellow keep fit teachers are frequently invited to put ratings, squaddies and aircrew through a full aerobic workout. Even the macho men in football and cricket have got the message too!

Nearly all of us have danced and some of us continue to. But what about sport and exercise?

When I left school 38 years ago, if you were seen in sports gear or, heaven forbid, a track-suit, you'd be marked out as some kind of nut-case – a jolly hockey sticks type who'd somehow never grown up. Women as a whole just didn't get involved in sport. Once we left school and got caught up in the hurly-burly of life it was the menfolk who went on to play active sports like football, rugby or cricket. Our closest contact with the game was shouting encouraging words from the touchline, making the teas and washing the dirty kit at the end of the day! Even if we'd bucked the trend, there were precious few leisure facilities for women around.

My, how things have changed! Today more than a third of the adult female population of Britain takes part in some sport or other. A survey by the Sports Council a few years back found that the most popular pursuit was swimming, closely followed by exercise to music and yoga.

That's one-third of the female population with some get up and go. But what about the other two-thirds? Among the many excuses the Sports Council heard was that hardy perennial "I haven't got time" and, intriguingly, "It'd wear my bones out and make them brittle." Now it's true that many women in middle-age are prone to brittle bone disease or osteoporosis, but it's completely untrue that exercise could bring it on. Far from it! We now know that load-bearing exercises like walking, running or dancing can increase bone density and positively avert the onset of this crippling disease. But more about that later.

Forget all the excuses – exercise is for all of us and it's fun. One of the great things about my career is travelling up and down the country and seeing the growth of exercise classes, particularly those designed for the more mature woman. There's many a 50-plus class I've seen where, contrary to expectations, they aren't gliding around to the strains of Victor Sylvester but bopping away to the latest top 20 hit!

And what do we get for all this exertion? A heck of a lot, I can tell you. Speaking for myself, I find that it gives me much more energy and stamina to cope with life's everyday problems. And now that the ridiculous notion of 'going for the burn' and feeling the pain have been banished from any self-respecting class, I feel exhilaration rather than exhaustion after a good work-out.

Besides exhilaration, I also feel four immediate benefits after exercising. And they all begin with **S**.

Firstly, there's **suppleness**, something we take for granted when we're young but need to work at as we get older. It's a really great feeling to be able to use our bodies efficiently and to be able to bend, stretch and reach to our full potential.

Secondly, there's **stamina** – that's being able to sustain free bodily movement for the length of time we need without feeling puffed, exhausted or faint. Exercise tones up our circulation and digestion as well as improving the way our hearts and lungs work.

Then there's **strength** – building strong muscles throughout the body to improve our shape and maintain a good posture. Strong muscles make light work of those everyday chores.

Finally there's **skill** – the natural co-ordination of mind and body, making your movements graceful, effective and efficient.

The average person would probably benefit from improving each of the four **S**'s in their lives. Athletes and competitive sportsmen and women would probably tend to concentrate more on stamina and strength. But that's one of the secrets of successful exercising – we all have individual aims and needs. And don't forget, we were all made differently. There really is no such thing as the perfect figure. Being slim doesn't necessarily mean being fit. Nature never intended us to carry pounds of excess baggage around our tums but neither did she turn us out on a production line, expecting us all to slip comfortably into a size eight! If we aim too high and expect the impossible we're bound to be disappointed and it's odds on we'll just give up.

The trick is to start slowly and gradually build up. You'll be amazed how soon you'll find you're able to achieve more. Once you get into the swing of things, take any opportunity you can to exercise a little more. A couple of minutes at home or in the office, in the back garden or on the beach, will make all the difference. Try to learn to be aware of your posture and your breathing. And as long as you keep up the good work, you'll find that it'll only take a month or so for your body to feel more supple and coordinated. But you must keep at it!

Remember too that exercise alone doesn't make us slim. True, a full aerobic work-out will attack some of the fat, tone up lazy muscles and improve the outline. But the only way to lose weight effectively is to watch what you eat and

T O P T I P

Eat plenty of fresh fruit and vegetables, and make the most of your freezer to store produce that would cost a king's ransom out of season!

drink. It's back to those principles I learnt all those years ago. The keys to success are exercise and nutrition.

More on diet later. But now a word on a peculiar form of vegetable that's entered the language over the past few years – the couch potato.

The couch potato is an unenviable fellow human being who spends most of his or her time slumped in an armchair., inevitably glued to the television, not only oblivious of what's on the screen, but equally oblivious of their ever-increasing waist-line and the feebleness of the rest of their body – and their mind for that matter!

Now sitting is something we all do naturally. It's good for us occasionally to 'take the weight off our feet'. But sitting down for too long can be positively harmful. Hours spent sitting at an office desk, in a car or couch potato-like in the privacy of our own home, slow down the heart. Our circulation becomes sluggish and the heart weakens.

Add to that the risk of varicose veins, back problems, stomach disorders and agonising cramp and you'd never look at a seat again! If you sit too long you'll also find yourself feeling tense and imagine that the whole weight of the world's problems seem to be bearing down on you. You get fuzzy and muzzy. But relief's at hand. How about a nice sugary drink, a bite or two of chocolate and maybe a glass or two of your favourite tipple to console yourself? Then you can slump back and start on the downward spiral all over again.

Far better to get up off your bottom and do something about your life! Our bodies were designed to walk, run, stretch and bend. It's just plain silly not to do anything about it. The fact that you're reading this book at least shows you're on the right track. But if you need any further encouragement just think what the penalties are for being overweight and out of condition. The tell-tale signs are obvious. You feel uncomfortable, you get out of breath, you're permanently tired and listless, a wet lettuce with nowhere to go. Your insides are even worse off than you feel. The circulation's poor, the blood pressure is up and the heart's at risk from disease. Rheumatism and arthritis are waiting in the wings and bad posture is inviting stomach problems. All in all, it's pretty depressing. You can't even get clothes that will fit and you're fed up. So back you go to a couple of chocolate bars, a drink or two and ...

Stop! It's time to get up and do something about yourself and the life you live.

But be honest with yourself. And as I've said before, set yourself an achievable goal. When it comes to your own body, you'll know best.

So, assuming you're on your own, strip off and take a long hard look at yourself in the mirror. Did nature, and by that I mean what you've inherited from your mother and father, intend you to look the way you do today? Probably not. All too many of us are overweight and carrying excess baggage in all the wrong places. And if you don't feel happy with what you see, you could certainly benefit from easing into fitness.

But first, a word or two about what we're planning to do.

Biologists break down our lives into four stages. In the first, from our birth to our teens, we are dependent on others. It's a time for education and development when *we* must learn and prepare ourselves for our lives ahead.

In our second age, the 20s, 30s and 40s, it's time for caring and sharing. For some of us, this means buckling down to the rigours of a job. Or it can mean taking on the responsibilities of running a home and bringing up demanding young children. For many of us, it can be a combination of both – and a particularly frustrating time it can be too!

The third age, the late 40s, 50s and 60s, is a time of liberation – a time when we may be set free from the constraints of our second age and can, at last, become ourselves and do what we want to do. These aren't bonus years, by the way,

TOP TIP

Don't drench your food in dressings, sauces, or salad creams. Try making your own low-fat dressings instead, or top your food with natural yogurt or low-fat fromage frais.

but quality time which we've not only earned but have spent our lives preparing for.

The fourth and final age, which of course varies from one individual to another, can be just as rewarding as the third. If we prepare and take care of ourselves, and are spared illness, then there is no reason to fall into the dependency that marked our first age.

Today, more than a fifth of the population is over 60. Not so long ago, life after 60 might have seemed a bleak prospect – 'How much longer have I got and who's going to look after me?' Now, thankfully, an increasing number are able to look ahead with optimism and ask 'How can I continue enjoying myself?'

But, as in all things in this life, a little bit of homework and preparation makes answering that question positively much more likely. If we've prepared during our second and third age and developed a healthy life-style by middle age then we're well on the road to success.

Upon reflection, I suppose that's what I did when I was 30. But at 40 most of us still have half our lives ahead of us. With care and attention we can look forward to being fitter and sounder than we were in youth. It is possible, you know!

My body and yours are the most complex machines in the world. Nothing that man has invented or is ever likely to invent will compare with the infinite possibilities of our minds and bodies. But if we do liken the body to a simple machine like a car, then one thing becomes blindingly obvi-ous. All cars benefit from being regularly checked and serviced. Tuning up improves performance and the right fuel and lubricants make it function as a well-oiled machine. Our bodies are just the same. The only differences are that unlike cars, which have a limit on how much fuel they can take, our bodies have no automatic cut-out and our sleek body-lines may just get fatter and fatter; neither, sadly, can we trade our bodies in for a new model when the rust begins to show!

From my experience, women are much more health-conscious than men. We tend to worry about our weight, and the magazines we read are full of this diet and that. We also buy more vitamin supplements and pursue alternative medicine with enthusiasm. But we continue to lag behind the menfolk when it comes to exercise. We've all heard and perhaps used the excuses – "I'm too tired" – "Not enough time" – 'Who's going to look after the children'.

The excuses sound pretty good – I used them myself once. But the effect on our bodies is no good at all. Careful eating and a balanced intake of vitamins are vital. But being fit is much more. It's the combination of a healthy diet *and* healthy exercise that's the key.

In the 1980s, as television's Green Goddess, I'm proud to have introduced tens of thousands to the idea of regular exercise. Now it's time to build on all the good work and help people find the combination of diet and exercise they need for a truly healthy life.

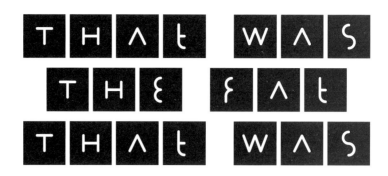

THAT WAS THE FAT THAT WAS

We are what we eat. Of course eating is one of life's pleasures but it's also a necessity. We need food to give us energy.

How much energy we need depends on the life we lead. But it's true to say that our parents and grandparents needed more to cope with the physical demands made on them. In their days they were positively encouraged to eat to 'keep up their strength'. And by golly they needed to! Just take a look round a modern kitchen and you'll see what I mean. Labour-saving devices have taken the sheer hard slog out of everyday life. Most men, too, are on to a cushy number. They probably drive to work where the most physical demanding task might be switching on the computer terminal.

Half a century ago there was good reason for encouraging people to eat more meat, eggs, butter, cheese and milk. They all produced fat, and it was fat that was needed to keep us going or at least keep warm during the winter in a house without central heating. Even then, of course, some people got *too* fat. The standard words of advice then were cut down on things like bread and potatoes – indeed, precisely the opposite of what they should have been told. And you'll soon understand why.

But first, we need to know more about the food we eat. The **energy** content of food is measured in **calories**. Ideally we should eat enough calories to go about our normal daily tasks, leaving just a little bit over for the body to use for growth and repairs.

The bread and potatoes which were shunned by our parents' generation are in fact rich in **carbohydrates**. Carbohydrates release their calorie content slowly, or to put it another way, they give us the bulk we need for a satisfying meal and then maintain our energy level over a long period.

Beware though of sugars – anything ending in 'ose', like sucrose, fructose or lactose. These are packed full of calories, but without the bulk of carbohydrates, they deceive the body and leave us wanting to eat more.

But the real villains in our everyday diet are **fats**, though even here, there are important differences. The worst of the bunch are the **saturated fats**. You'll find these in red meats such as beef, lamb and pork. They're also in dairy products such as full-cream milk and cheese and in suet, lard and dripping. The calorie content is sky-high and so too is the cholesterol level – a dangerous fat that clogs the arteries and increases the risk of heart disease or failure.

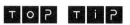

Buy semi-skimmed milk rather than full cream. It's far less fattening. And if, like me, you've a sweet tooth, kick the sugar bowl out of the kitchen and go for artificial sweeteners.

On the other hand, **unsaturated fats** are much more healthy. You'll find them in vegetable oils and margarines such as sunflower, corn, soya, rape seed and olive. They're also in oily fish like pilchards, herrings, mackerel, sardines and tuna. Great to eat and good for you!

So much for the theory. But what are we really supposed to do about it?

The answer is to learn but to stop worrying! Mention 'diet' to most people and their immediate thought is of some awful regime of rabbit food, or even worse, a ghastly concoction of powders, tablets and anonymous liquids. It sounds like a nightmare of starvation and anyone in their right mind would run a mile. That's if you could!

Hard cheeses like Cheddar and Stilton are packed full of calories. If you're a cheesy, choose Edam, Camembert or Cottage Cheese, or look out for your old favourites with reduced fat.

What I mean by diet is something completely different. If we learn about the plus and minus points of food we like, then far from suffering, we should positively enjoy what we eat, pick and mix our favourites and set ourselves on the road to a fitter and leaner self.

What we're looking for is more of the **F**'s and less of the **S**'s. The F's are fibre, fruit and vegetables. And the S's are sugar and salt. More about fibre in a moment. But back to the F we can positively do without, or at least cut down on: fats.

Do try to cut down on saturated fats. Go for poultry and fish rather than red meats. But if temptation gets the upper hand, do at least cut off the excess fat before cooking. Grill rather than fry. And be aware that sausages and burgers are probably more full of fat and stodge than anything else.

Also watch out for the dairy products. Skip the butter and hard cheese like cheddar and choose polyunsaturated margarines or low-fat cheeses. Milk, on the other hand, is a valuable source of protein and calcium for healthy bones and teeth. But don't buy full-cream. Go for semi-skimmed or skimmed. The calcium and protein levels are equally high but semi-skimmed tastes just as good although some people find skimmed tastes a little thin.

Beware, too, of all the products that lurk on supermarket shelves that are full of hidden fats – crisps, biscuits, cakes, pastries, and that old devil, chocolate.

Now, a final word on fats and a word of warning about that inevitable family favourite – chips. Chips are, all said and done, potatoes. And we already know that potatoes are rich in carbohydrates. But sloppy frying increases the calorie content of our humble spud three-fold. And if you cook in lard, well.... The trick with chips is to think of them as a special treat. On high days and holidays cook them thick and straight, not thin and serrated. That way, they'll soak up less oil. Choose a polyunsaturated oil and only immerse them when it's really hot. Once they're out of the frier, drain them on kitchen paper to blot away any excess fat. Alternatively, but again not too often, try oven-baked chips. They taste just as good and contain far less fat.

So much for the humble spud – just one of the many sources of valuable carbohydrates. Valuable not only

TOP TIP

If you're a meat eater, go for poultry or fish. Red meats like beef, lamb or pork are full of saturated fats that not only fatten us up but increase the risk of heart disease. And do throw away your frying pan. Grilling is great!

because of their energy content, but also because they are usually filling, not too high in calories and relatively inexpensive.

Many of the sources of carbohydrates are also rich in **fibre**; things like cereals, beans, peas, most fruit, grains, and seeds. You'll find a high fibre content too in wholemeal bread, wholegrain pasta and brown rice. Eating these is not only satisfying, they can also tone up the digestion, giving you regular bowel movements and helping to avoid constipation. On top of these benefits, oats, beans, fruit and vegetables contain a type of fibre which is believed to help reduce the amount of cholesterol in the bloodstream.

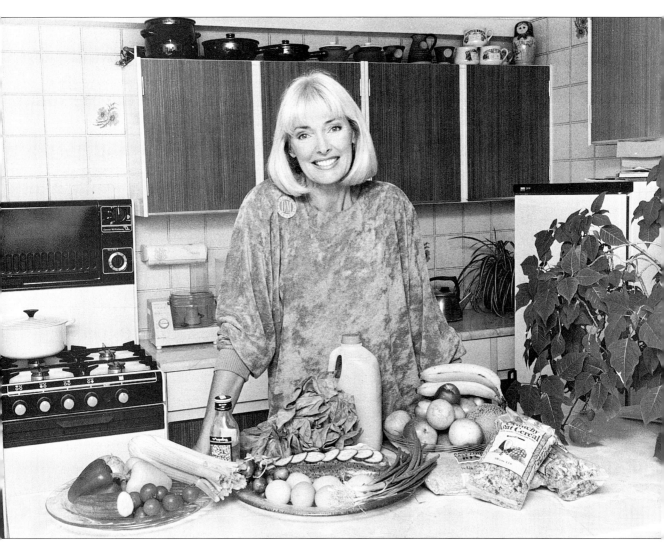

Keep temptation out of sight. Store biscuits, chocolates and cakes in tins or opaque containers so you're not tempted to binge. Better still, don't buy them in the first place!

If, like me, you choose a diet that's rich in fibre, then a word of advice and a word of warning. Firstly, it's important to drink enough fluids every day to help flush out the system. Aim to drink at least six pints a day – a mixture of water, tea, decaffeinated coffee, fruit juices and so on, with the emphasis on water.

Secondly, if you haven't previously eaten much fibre, take things easily at first. Otherwise the results can be uncomfortable and you'll become the victim of wind! Far better to start simply by eating more potatoes and their skins, either boiled as new potatoes or in their jackets. Don't smother them in butter though! You could also choose brown rice rather than white – it's full of fibre and a lot more tasty. Most breakfast cereals are also good fibre providers, but the less processed the better. And certainly avoid those that have been coated in sugar or honey. Later on in the day, peas, beans, and lentils are easy to prepare and can form the basis of a delicious meal. And a firm favourite for most of us is a tin of baked beans – cheap both to buy and to cook, and packed full of fibre. But go for the reduced sugar versions that virtually all the manufacturers have now introduced.

Sugar really isn't necessary if we're eating a well-balanced and nutritious diet. Sugar is just like a quick fix. It kids the body it's getting the energy but all too often all it's doing is bumping up the calorie intake and leaving us wobbling down the primrose path to obesity. Sugary foods like cakes, pastries and chocolate also contain large amounts of fat, fattening for sure, and more than likely to cause tooth decay, particularly in children.

As I've said before, anything ending in 'ose' is a sugar by another name, so it's well worth taking the time to read the labels on the food you buy. Indeed, once you've set out on the path to healthy eating, you'll find the manufacturers' information not only useful and revealing, but sometimes positively frightening! If you have got the dreaded sweet tooth, then you can easily cut down on your sugar intake by using artificial sweeteners in tea or coffee and buying low calorie soft drinks and fruit juices.

The other S, salt, is also a regular and unwelcome guest on manufacturers' labels. Processed foods such as crisps, peanuts and nibbles, canned vegetables, ham, bacon and salted fish have all had salt added, either for taste or preservative reasons. All such foodstuffs contribute to our vast over-eating of salt. Our bodies only need one gram a day. On average though our daily intake is ten times that amount. And it's a sad fact that excess salt can cause high blood pressure, heart disorders and strokes. So whatever you do, banish the salt cellar from the dining table. You just don't need it.

Fortunately, the message about healthy eating is beginning to get through to the public at large and the traditional – and disastrous – British diet is changing. According to the most recent figures from the Ministry of Agriculture, we're eating less dairy produce. Consumption of milk and cream is down by a fifth and we're also down to a third of our previous intake of butter. Strangely, though, there's been an increase in the consumption of cheese. Hens can rest easy too – our consumption of eggs is down by a third. Maybe it's time for belated thanks to Edwina Currie! Our sugar intake is also down by a half and meat eaters have cut back by a sixth.

On the positive side, we're eating more healthy fruit and vegetables and drinking more fruit juices. But somehow the message about potatoes and bread still hasn't got through. Nutritionists are still finding it an uphill struggle to persuade us that these products, along with pasta and wholegrain rice, are positively good for us. The misconceptions of the past were based not on the simple foods themselves but the way we ruined them. Lashings of jam and butter on bread, and fat-fried chips, pushed our calorie intake sky-high. Indeed, despite all the warnings we still

TOP TIP

When you're out shopping, always buy fresh food rather than processed if you can. Manufactured products that sit on the shelf are almost certainly full of sugars, fats and salts that you can do without.

TOP TIP

Remember that soft drinks can often be sky-high in calories. Watch out for sugary squashes and minerals. Drink natural fresh fruit juice instead.

seem addicted to fat, as the rise in the consumption of cakes and biscuits so readily proves.

Before we leave food, I'd just like to put the record straight on one thing. It's all too easy to condemn the average diet of our parents' and grandparents' generations. But, as I've already said, their nutritional needs were very different from our own. And perhaps more importantly, they didn't have the choice of foods that we have today.

Most preserved food 40 or 50 years ago was salted, canned or dried. It was still possible, as my mother ably proved, to make the most of dried fruit, pulses and lentils. But fresh fruit or vegetables, out of season, were beyond the reach of all but the very rich, and milk was milk – even that awful lukewarm offering that we all had to endure during morning break at school! Thank you, whoever you were, to the person who dreamt up semi-skimmed milk, and thank goodness for the fridge!

Nowadays, virtually every supermarket and market stall in the land has seasonal fresh fruit and vegetables from all over the world. Buy them and enjoy them when they're plentiful and cheap. And if you've a particular favourite, make the most of your freezer and put some aside for later in the year. Incidentally, don't fall into the trap of being an anti-freezer snob. Most frozen food, like fish, peas and so on, has a much higher vitamin content than their so-called fresh counterparts that have been hanging around for a day or two on the shelf, waiting to be sold.

Next time you're out shopping, just take a careful look at what you're buying. If you're buying for a family, think too of their future health. Remember the **F**'s and the **S**'s and you won't go far wrong. Remember, too, to avoid processed foods. If you do buy them, take a good look at the manufacturer's list of ingredients and make a mental list of the calorie content. On average, women between 19 and 50 need 1,940 calories a day, men of the same age 2,550. And we need less as we grow older.

Above all, enjoy your food. Think of trading fried fish and chips for steamed fish, a large portion of boiled new potatoes, peas and sweetcorn. You'd still be way down the calorie count and be free to tuck into some fresh fruit and fromage frais afterwards. Much healthier and definitely more tasty!

It has never been easier to eat healthily and a well-balanced diet is the first vital step to a leaner and fitter self. For most of our lives we need nothing else. But sometimes we can do just a little bit more.

If you've been ill, are convalescing or pregnant, you may find that you need to take vitamin and mineral supplements. Iron is particularly important for women during pregnancy and can help during heavy periods and the menopause. You might find, too, that if you're on a strictly vegetarian or vegan diet that you need to take supplements. Consult your doctor or chemist and they will advise you. You'll also find plenty of helpful advice in the literature provided by the manufacturers.

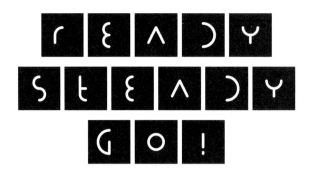

So you've tackled your diet, you're eating healthily and you're raring to go off in hot pursuit of those wonderful **S**'s, stamina, strength and suppleness. But hold on just a minute!

Exercise is not only good for you, it's also fun. But you shouldn't start out on this fresh path to fitness if you're currently in poor health, suffer from a bad back or joints, have a heart complaint, or are severely overweight or pregnant. If you're in any doubt, please check with your doctor before starting. It's better to be safe than sorry. It's also important to begin slowly and build up gradually. Listen to your body and don't overstrain. If it hurts, stop. Enhanced activity will become easier with practice. And finally, go at your own pace – you're not in a race with anyone.

Easing into fitness will mean different things to different people. Remember we're all made differently and we all have different goals and different expectations for ourselves. When you come to the exercises ahead you'll find it easy to pick and mix and choose just what *you* want to do. Ideally, though, your aim should be to do 20 minutes exercise at least three times a week but no more than six. It might seem an impossible dream now, but just you wait and see. A little bit of practice and you'll wonder what all the fuss was about.

Now, you're almost ready to go. But don't even think of exercising after a heavy meal. Leave at least an hour for your food to be digested.

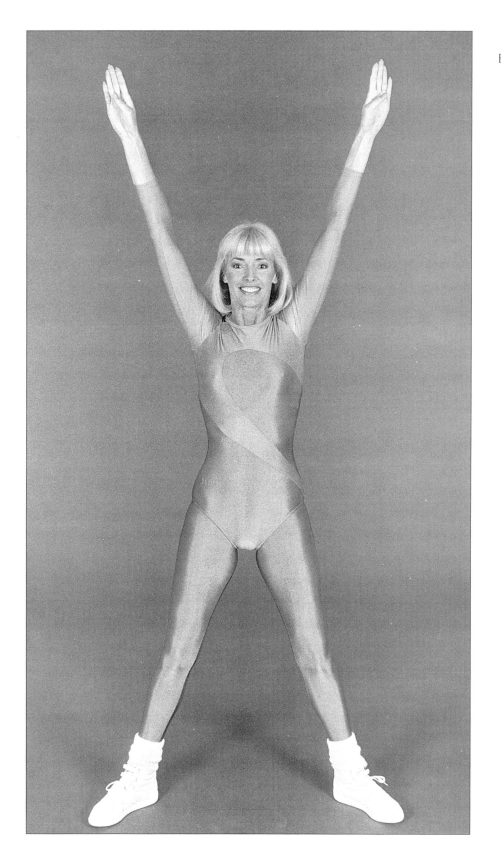

And what do you need to join in? Not a lot. Just loose comfortable clothing and some suitable shoes – trainers, like Reeboks, are the best. And of course you'll need to clear a space before you start!

But first, always remember to check your posture throughout the exercises. Stand with your feet comfortably apart. Pull your tummy in and tuck your bottom under. Keep your shoulders back, but down and relaxed. Keep your knees soft and relaxed too. We're not on the parade ground! And make sure your knees are in line over your toes when you bend. And if the exercises call for jogging or marching, make sure your heels come down – don't work on your toes.

And don't expect to be able to do everything perfectly the first time round. Take it slowly and surely and very soon you'll begin to feel the benefits of a regular work-out. Your body will become firmer, your skin will take on a healthy glow, your mind will be more relaxed and you'll find it easier to tackle and cope with everyday problems. It may sound like a miracle, but it's a fair reward for the hard work you'll have put in.

You'll also find that your breathing will improve. Don't worry if you find yourself panting a little during the Fat Attack (Aerobics) section. That's normal and good for you. Just breathe more deeply and fill your lungs with air – good fresh outdoor air is even better.

The only exercises that will help you lose weight, as their name suggests, are those in the Fat Attack section. These aerobic exercises require extra energy – energy which is stored in the body as unused and unwanted fat. Someone once said that middle age is when your age started to show round your middle! Sadly too true for too many. But an increase in years really is no excuse for an increase in inches around the waistline.

Don't worry either if you can't get all the way through the Fat Attack section of the exercise programme. Fitness comes with practice. But the exercises that call for gentle stretching really require very little effort – effort you'll soon find repaid in added flexibility.

Remember, all exercise is good for you. Once you've got into the swing of things you'll find regular exercise habit forming. And this is one habit you *don't* have to kick. And once you've got motivated, feel free to spread the word. You could even try to persuade family and friends to join in.

You're never too young to look after your diet and, likewise, never too old to start exercising. But do remember that you can't recapture your youth, and don't make the mistake of trying to keep up with the youngsters. It really is an unequal struggle. And don't worry either, particularly if you haven't exercised for years, if you feel a little stiff a day or so after you've exercised. As long as it's not extreme, think of it as an indication of the healthy effort you've put in. But keeping fit is not a competition. And don't believe the nonsense that there's no gain without pain. Pain has got nothing to do with fitness. If you do feel pain, it's more than likely that your body is crying out for you to stop.

Follow the exercise in this book or mirror my movements on my video, also called *Ease Into Fitness*, and you'll be doing fine. But don't stop there. Make the most of your local park and go for a brisk walk or maybe even a jog too. It will all help.

Learn to use your body more. Start walking to places which, in your bad old lazy days, you'd have reached by car or bus. If you can walk to the shops all the better. Carrying the shopping home, as long as it's not too heavy, is a beneficial exercise in itself. It'll also discourage you from buying things that you can do without! And when you're out shopping or at work, give the lifts or escalators a miss. Walking upstairs is a good natural exercise that will strengthen your leg muscles. If you've got a garden, make the most of it and tackle some of those chores that have been waiting around for ages. And if you're young at heart, why not have a go at disco-dancing? You'd be surprised how many grannies I've seen putting the youngsters to shame.

TOP TIP

Do exercise at least three times a week for at least 20 minutes. You don't have to head off for a gym or even follow my exercise routines (though I'd rather you did). Anything that makes you puff a bit and makes you work that little bit harder is better than nothing.

If you've got a bike, take Norman Tebbit's advice and get on it. Cycling is wonderful exercise for the lungs and legs and will improve stamina and strength and help maintain mobility. Swimming, too, is an excellent way to get fit and stay fit. With the body weight supported by water, it's ideal for anyone who is overweight or handicapped with a bad back or stiff joints. And it's a great improver of all three **S**'s, stamina, strength and suppleness.

Most importantly, don't be alarmed if, to begin with, you seem to be putting on weight rather than losing it. The muscles you are developing weigh more than flab and can add a pound or two. But not to worry. Keep an eye on your diet and get into the swing of our Fat Attack and you'll soon find the scales giving you the answer you want.

Incidentally, if you like to follow the latest fads and fashions, the craze that's sweeping the United States now is both cheap and cheerful. To put it bluntly, it's a good old-fashioned brisk walk. Hardly a new invention, but if you walk at a good pace, you'll find yourself panting a bit (taking in more fresh air) and your heart will be beating faster, bringing all-round benefit to your body. So go on, take the dog for a walk. You'll both benefit. If you haven't got a dog, buy a nice big one and let *him* take *you* for a walk!

Whatever activities you choose, try to involve your family and friends and you'll soon discover three other benefits that come from regular exercise – and they all begin with **F**. **Fitness**, **friendship** and **fun**.

Getting Better All The Time?

As I've said before, apart from illness and hereditary factors, fitness really is one of our most valuable birthrights. But it's still, sadly, a right that many of us are prepared to forego.

A recent survey on fitness by Allied Dunbar on behalf of the Health Education Authority and the Sports Council revealed some disturbing facts about the nation's health and our general lack of physical activity.

For instance, seven out of ten men and eight out of ten women were found to be doing less exercise than needed to improve their health.

Middle-aged men were found to be particularly lethargic, with four out of five of 45 to 54 year olds failing to achieve a sufficient level of exercise and risking potential heart disease.

Even more disturbing were the figures for the youngsters. Among 16 to 24 year olds, seven out of ten men and a staggering nine out of ten women fell below a target level of exercise that would actively improve their health.

At the other end of the age range, among the 65 to 74 year olds, three out of ten men and five out of ten women didn't even have enough muscular strength to get up from a chair without holding on to the arms. Leg power was also low among older women over 55, where five out of ten needed help to climb stairs.

Most disturbing of all was the discovery of how many of us kid ourselves that all's well. The survey found that 80 per cent of all ages, both men and women, believed they were as fit as they could be and already did enough exercise. There also appeared to be a general misunderstanding that you had to be a 'sporty type' to indulge in any further activity.

The report also highlighted how different our lives are today compared with, say thirty or forty years ago. It concluded that 80 per cent of men and 90 per cent of women no longer work in vigorous or moderately vigorous occupations. It's small wonder that fitness professionals such as myself take our jobs so seriously and never fail to bang the drum!

On the flab front, the report found that the number of people overweight appears to be increasing. In 1980, 39 per cent of men and 32 per cent of women were found to be overweight. Today the figures are 48 per cent of men and

40 per cent of women. Eight per cent of men and 13 per cent of women were considered to be obese.

Sadly, too, the dreaded male 'beer belly' seems to be gaining ground. Among middle-aged men, 11 per cent had waist measurements that were larger than their hip size. Such body fat puts them at real risk of heart disease.

On the positive side, the report indicated that participation in sport or exercise reduces the risk of heart disease, angina and breathlessness. And smoking got the real thumbs down it deserves with those who smoked more than 20 a day being found to be substantially less active than their non-smoking counterparts.

FIT FOR WHAT?

Enough of statistics. Now for a little science. But don't worry, it's nothing too complicated, just an insight into the complex but truly miraculous machinery of our bodies.

It goes without saying that our bodies rely on our hearts and lungs. We take oxygen in through the lungs where it is dissolved into the bloodstream. Oxygenated blood is then circulated throughout the body by the pumping action of the heart, passes through the arteries and returns for re-oxygenation via the veins.

All our muscles require oxygen to function properly and convert carbohydrates and fats into the energy we expend in physical activity. Converting food into energy is the basic mechanism of metabolism. Even this simplest of explanations shows how vital to our well-being our hearts and lungs are. We also refer to them as our cardiovascular system. Through exercise, and aerobic exercise in particular, we aim to strengthen our hearts and lungs, enabling them to work more efficiently. A strong heart will pump more blood per beat and with increased efficiency it also reduces the pulse rate when we're at rest and helps reduce the risk of high blood pressure.

Exercise also speeds up the efficiency of the circulation and helps it deliver what the body needs and removes waste products more effectively. In simple terms, exercise peps up the system.

As I've said, muscles need energy for action. But there are two forms of action and two forms of energy. The first sort of action is the one that calls for immediate energy – an instantaneous reaction to stimulus, probably lasting only five to ten seconds. Dashing to catch a bus or grabbing a falling child are good examples of this.

Such action calls upon **phosphate** or **anaerobic** energy. Anaerobic means 'without air' and is also know as **glycogen** energy after the complex carbohydrate from which it is derived. You can look upon it as the body's back up system in times of emergency. Glycogen is also stored in the liver where it can be called upon to fuel longer bursts of energy – the sort needed by sprinters or footballers speeding for the goal, or indeed by any of us who suddenly up the pace.

But unfortunately there's a price to pay for this energy. Whenever we call upon the body to convert glycogen energy into muscle power, we're also creating lactic acid. As this by product builds up it makes us feel tired, even exhausted, and our muscles feel sore. With such discomfort, it's no surprise that we soon give up and stop the activity that produces this effect. For more sustained periods of activity we call upon a different form of energy, and one that is much more familiar to us these days – aerobic energy. During aerobic ('with air') exercise oxygen reaches the muscles which in turn draw upon the body's reserves of fat, breaking this down to fuel their sustained activity. Unlike anaerobic energy and its build up of lactic acid, aerobic energy produces no unpleasant side-effects and has the beneficial effect of burning off the excess calories stored in the body as fat. Fortunately, aerobic energy is the main source we use in our everyday lives, and our fitness training should be designed to increase our aerobic capacity.

The more capacity, the more we will be able to keep going at work and play. Or, to put it another way, the fitter we will be. Anyone who is unfit and makes the mistake of trying to keep up with us will be calling on their anaerobic system with the inevitable consequence of exhaustion, pain and failure.

Fit for Anything

You're now within a stone's throw of embarking on your own fitness plan – one that's purpose-designed to build up your aerobic capacity slowly and surely. But until you understand the difference between aerobic and anaerobic, you will not see why I constantly stress the need to take things gradually. Go at your own pace and you'll soon find that you've all the energy you need to climb the stairs, take a brisk walk, indeed work *and* play without becoming tired, out of breath, or mentally or physically exhausted.

Take things too quickly, and far from feeling 'full of beans' you are more than likely to make yourself feel moody and irritable.

No, fitness should enable us to face the future optimistically, to take everything in our stride and assure us of a full and satisfying life, full of zest and energy – a life too where our chances of serious illness are substantially reduced, and one in which we can call upon our bodies rather than a packet of pills to keep ourselves going.

By the way, you don't have to keep going all the time! But when you're fit you'll find you'll not only sleep sounder, you'll also wake up feeling bright, lively and raring to go!

Surely this is all the motivation you could need to **ease into fitness**?

Build up your own personal exercise programme, always aiming at a target you know is within your reach, and you'll find that exercise will relieve tension, lift depression, see you through a mid-life crisis – all in all, make you look and feel like a member of the human race who positively glows with health.

One final tip, and one final word of warning. The tip is – **don't forget your diet!** The warning is, **don't expect miracles**. If you're out of condition and carrying some excess fat, you've almost certainly built it up over quite a long period of time. Plan to lose just a couple of pounds a week and you will be on the right track. Certainly there are hundreds of so-called instant diets on the market that will achieve a much quicker weight loss. But in effect, almost all of them are simply fooling your body into thinking it's starving. Your metabolism slows down and the body does its utmost to conserve as much fat as possible. The apparent loss is mostly in fluids, just a little fat, and a certain amount of muscle. It might look convincing on the scales, but your system will be all over the place. You'll feel weaker and be a ripe candidate to go zooming up the scales again as soon as your guard is down.

Do it my way. Ease into fitness, by taking it steady and going all the way.

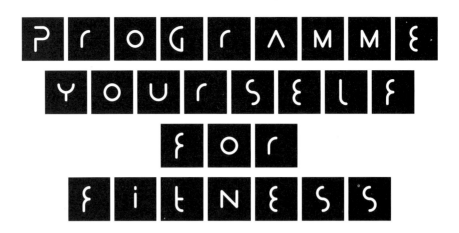

PROGRAMME YOURSELF FOR FITNESS

THE WARM UP

In the Warm Up our aim is to motivate and mobilise the body by going through a specific range of movements, to wake up the body and the mind and encourage co-ordination. The exercise will mobilise the major joints by taking them through their full range of movement. In the process, synovial fluid will be released to lubricate the joints and 'free us up'. As the body gets warmer, so too do the muscles. And warm muscles prevent soreness and possible injury during the more strenuous Fat Attack work-out to follow. Initially the movements are precise and are aimed at specific joints but as the warm up progresses, movements will become larger and our pulse rate should start to quicken.

Whatever exercise you choose to do, don't forget you should always warm up first, and always go to the Relax and Stretch exercises at the end of your work-out.

The reason I, like most teachers of exercise, wear leotards and tights instead of baggy clothes is in order to demonstrate correct technique and body alignment to enable you to copy my movement safely and effectively.

TOP TIP

*Drink a lot. **No, not alcohol!** Your body needs six pints of water a day to flush out the system. And make sure you don't dehydrate when you're exercising.*

Check Your Posture

Stand up tall with your feet comfortably hip width apart and your weight evenly distributed over both feet. Your knees should be 'soft' (not flexed) and they should be in line over your toes.

Pull in your abdominal (tummy) muscles, clench the muscles of your bottom and tuck it under, and tilt your pelvis forward. Check that your shoulders are back but down and relaxed. Hold your head up and lift your chin so that it is parallel to the ground not facing it.

Make your warm up last for between 10-15 minutes. The less fit you are, the longer you will need to warm up. All your movements should be rhythmic, not jerky. If you do these exercises to music of a medium speed, it will help you.

1 *To Mobilise the Shoulder Joints*
Lift alternate shoulders to ear level and press back down again. Don't take ears to shoulders.

8 repetitions.

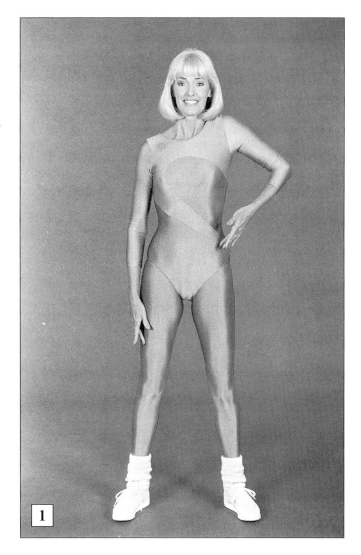

2 *To Mobilise the Shoulder Joints*

Lift both of your shoulders slowly forward and up. Circle them on back down and around, pulling your shoulder-blades together.

4 repetitions forward, 4 repetitions backwards.

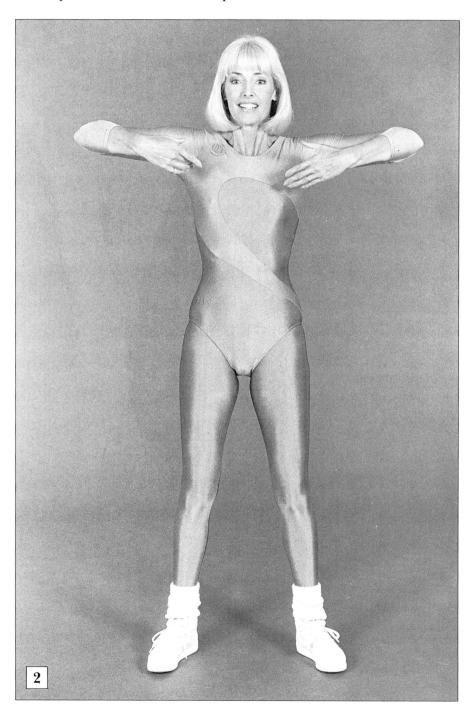

2

3 *To Mobilise Your Ankles and Feet*

Place one foot out in front, heel to floor. Bring your foot back, touch toes to side of your other foot. Repeat heel/toe action, keeping supporting leg 'soft'.

8 repetitions each side.

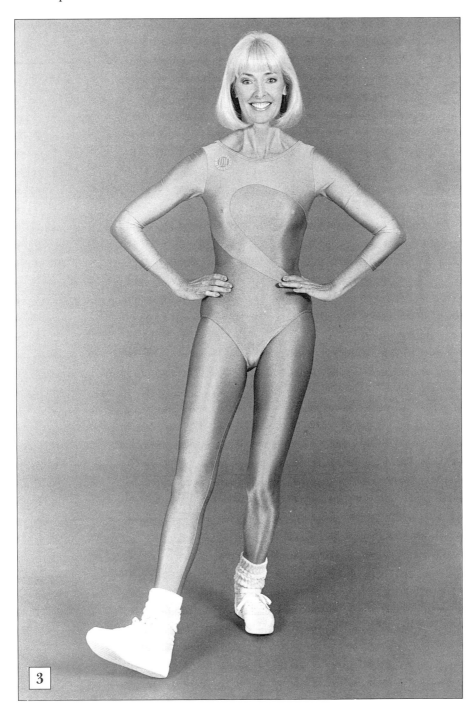

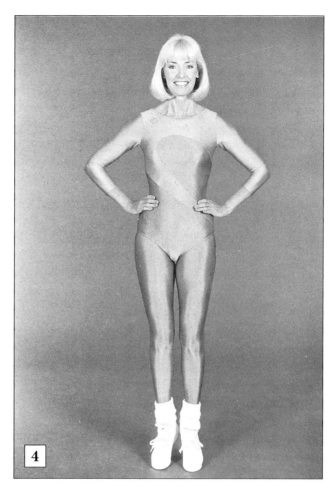

4 *To Mobilise Your Ankles and Feet*

Stand with your feet comfortably apart, toes facing forward. Slowly rise up on to your toes and then lower. Remember your posture, and don't allow your feet to roll in or out at the ankles. Keep your weight over the big toe (you could use a chair for support).

8 repetitions.

5 *To Mobilise Your Knees and Hips*

Stand with your feet wider apart, and toes turned out. Keep your heels down and bend your knees out, keeping them in line with your toes. Back straight, tummy tight, bottom under. Again you could use a chair for support. Only go down as far as comfortable.

8 repetitions.

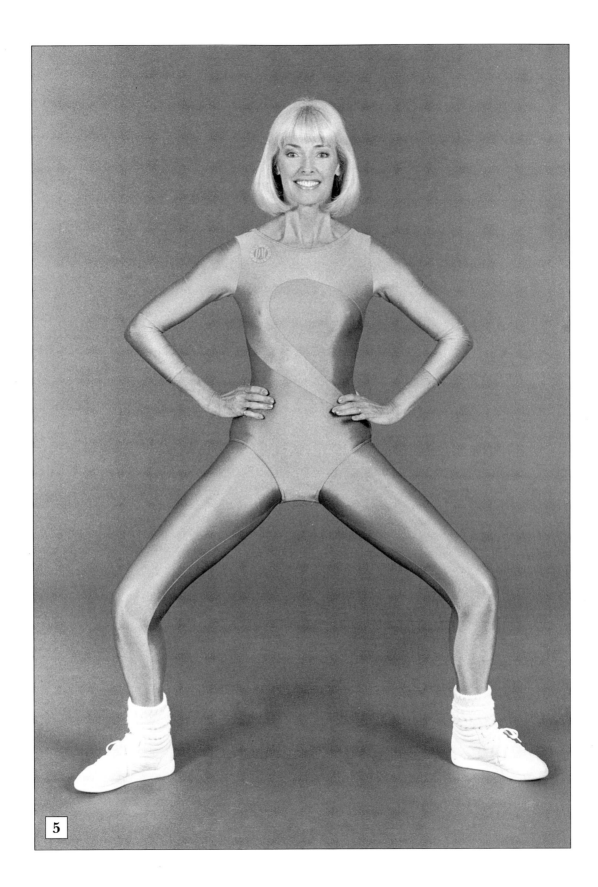

5

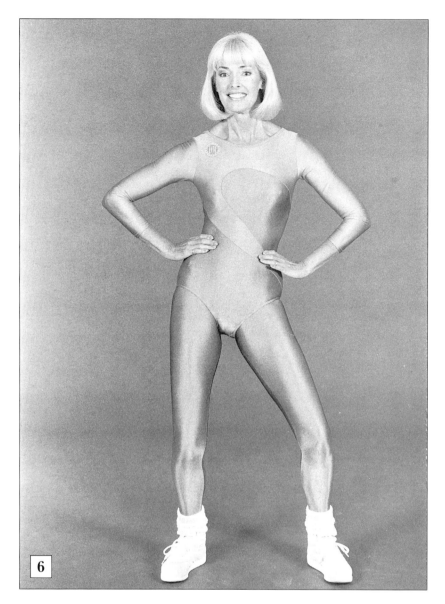

6

6 *To Mobilise the Hips*

Stand with hips shoulder width apart. Pull your tummy in and keep your bottom tight. Keeping your upper body steady, swing your hips in a controlled motion from side to side.

8 repetitions.

Now slowly 'circle' your hips 4 times in a clockwise direction. Repeat anti-clockwise.

Now tilt your pelvis slowly forward and up and back, taking care not to 'arch' your back.

8 repetitions.

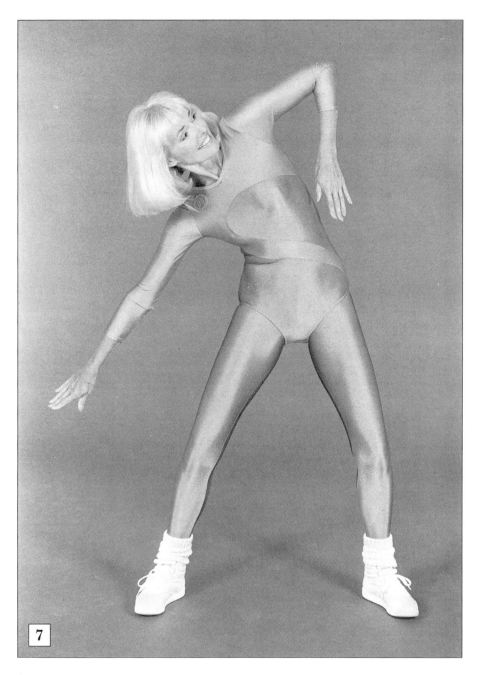

7 *To Mobilise the Sides of Your Body and to Raise the Pulse*
Stand upright with your feet wider apart. Remember your
posture and keep your knees soft. Keep your hips facing
forward, lead with your arm and take your head and upper
body over to one side. Slowly come back to the centre and
bend to the other side. Don't lean forwards or backwards.

4 repetitions each side.

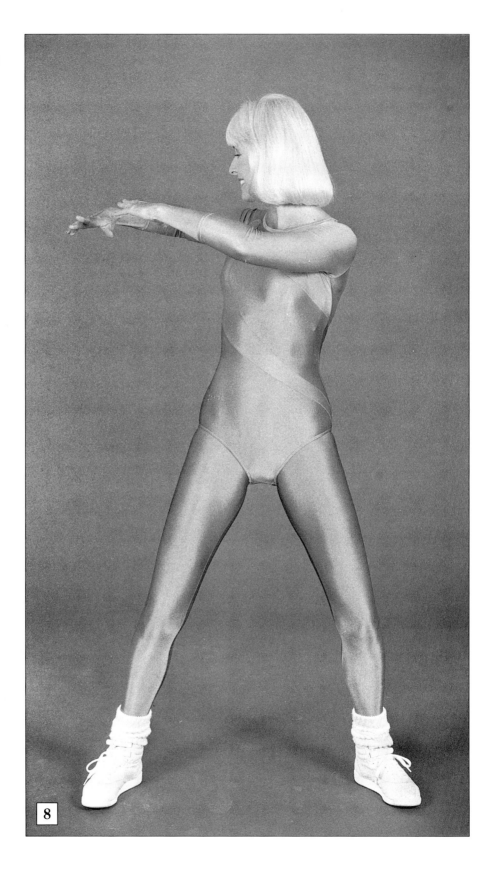

8

8 *To Mobilise Your Upper Body and Raise Your Pulse*

Stand as before, arms up and out to the front at shoulder level. Keeping your hips facing the front, twist only your upper body and arms around and look first to one side, back to centre, and on round to the other side.

4 repetitions each side.

9

From the same position, reach alternate arms up and over your head as if you were picking apples. Keep your knees soft and don't bend forwards or backwards.

8 repetitions.

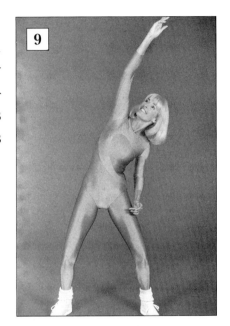

10

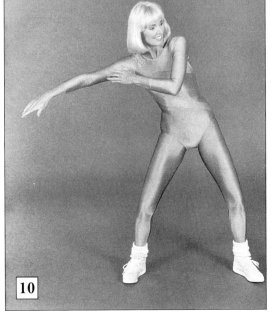

With your feet still further apart, bend your knees and transfer your weight from one foot to the other as you rhythmically swing your arms down and across your body and up high to either side. Remember your posture and don't bend over and forward from your waist.

8 repetitions.

Build up the repetitions of these warm up exercises until your joints feel easy and your body warm.

WARM UP STRETCHES

Hold all these preparation stretches for 8 seconds

11 *Calf Stretch*

Stand with one foot, toes facing forward. Bend the knee and take the other foot back behind you. With the knee straight, place it hip width apart, toes facing forward and push your heel down. If need be, take the foot back still further until you feel the stretch in your calf. Remember your posture and keep your body upright.

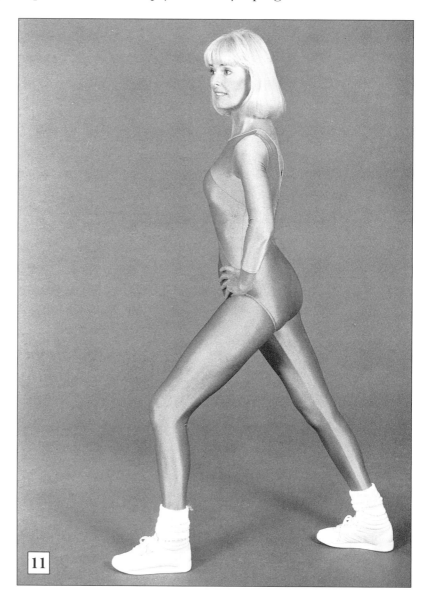

11

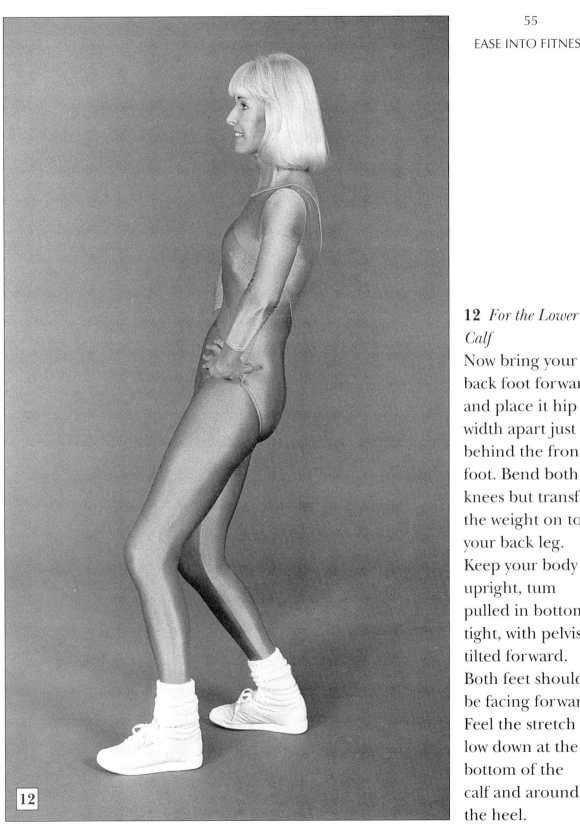

12

12 *For the Lower Calf*
Now bring your back foot forward and place it hip width apart just behind the front foot. Bend both knees but transfer the weight on to your back leg. Keep your body upright, tum pulled in bottom tight, with pelvis tilted forward. Both feet should be facing forward. Feel the stretch low down at the bottom of the calf and around the heel.

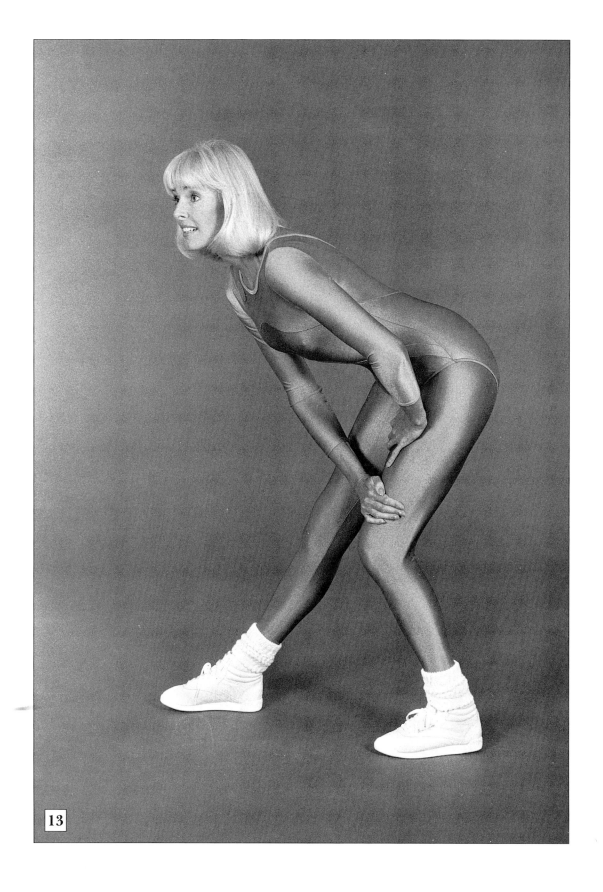

13 *For the Hamstrings*

Move the same leg again and place it in front with the foot facing forward and knee straightened out. Place your hands on the thigh of your other leg (bend the knee). Lift your bottom up on the side of the straight leg and feel the stretch in the hamstring (back of thigh).

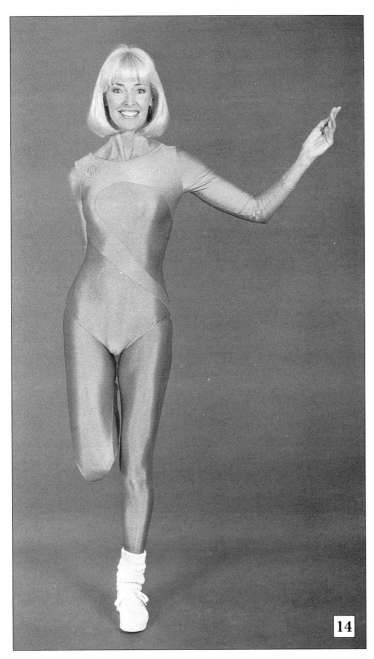

14 *For the Quadriceps (Front of Thigh)*
Stand with your feet together, one arm out to your side for balance. Take your other arm around and grasp your ankle on the same side and ease your foot towards your bottom. Keep both front thighs parallel and feel the stretch in the front of your thighs. Only bring your knees together if it is comfortable.

Repeat these four stretches for the other leg.

15 *For Your Upper Back*
Remember your
posture and keep
your knees soft.
Clasp both hands out
in front of your chest,
round out and feel
the stretch across
your upper back.

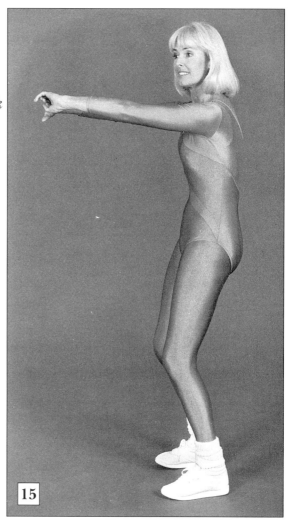

16 *For Your Pectorals (Chest)*
From the same position take your arms behind you and
clasp your hands together. Pull back your shoulders and feel
the stretch across your chest. But don't arch your back.

17 *For Your Triceps (Upper Arms)*
Take one hand up behind you and place it behind your
neck, fingers facing down. Take your other hand over your
head and use it to ease the elbow back until you feel
a stretch in your upper arm. If this is too difficult, simply
take your arm across your chest instead to ease your arm
gently back. Repeat with your other arm.

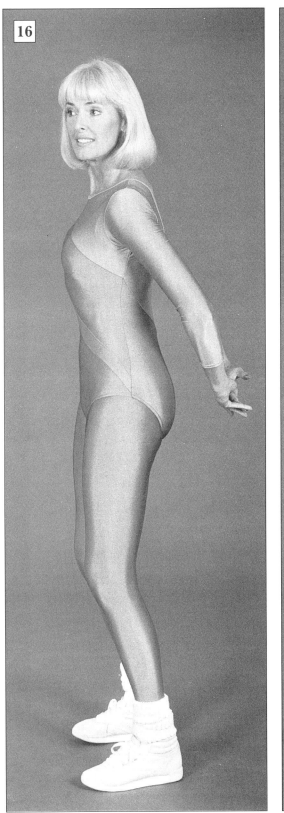
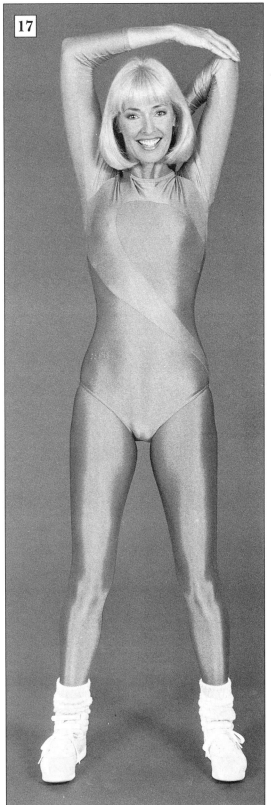

18

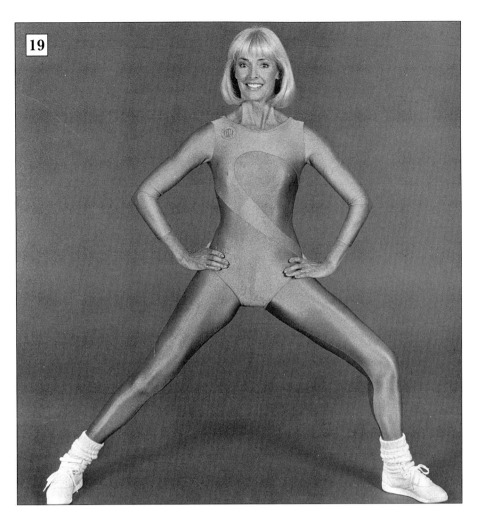

18 *For the sides of Your Body*
Stand with your feet wide apart. Place one hand on your thigh, bend your knees and with your other arm, reach up and over your head. Hold, and feel the stretch in your side. Don't bend forward or backward. Repeat for your other side.

19 *For the Abductors (Inner Thigh)*
Feet still further apart with one foot facing diagonally forward and your knee bent and in line with your toes. Straighten and take your other leg still wider apart, placing your foot flat on the floor with your toes facing forward. Keep your hips facing forward and your body upright. Hands on the bent knee for support. Feel the stretch in the inner thigh of the straight leg. Repeat to the other side. (It may be necessary to move the feet still wider apart to feel the stretch.)

20 *For the Groin*

Stand with your feet wide apart and turned out on a diagonal. Pull your tum in, tuck your tail under and tilt your pelvis forward. Bend and keep both knees over the toes and 'sit down' between your legs. Keep your back straight and feel the stretch in your groin.

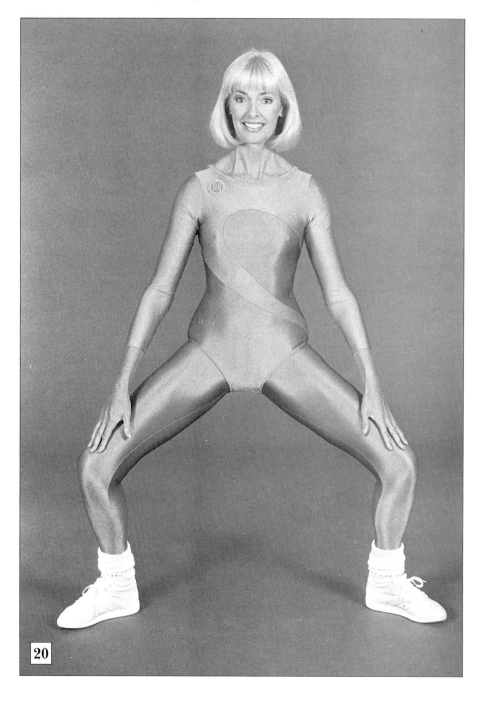

20

21 *For Your Neck*

Sit or stand comfortably and take your head over with the ear towards your shoulder. Hold for 8 seconds and repeat to the other side. Now drop your chin to your chest and hold. Carefully take your head back (but only if it is comfortable) and pull up your jaw. Feel the stretch under your chin.

Keep breathing easily throughout all these stretches.

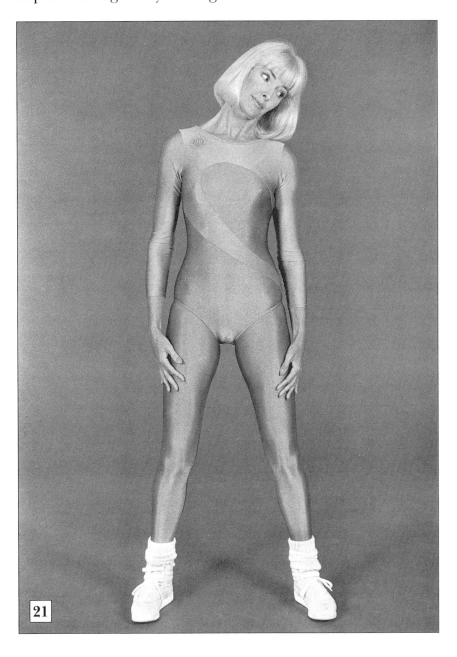

21

FAT ATTACK (AEROBICS)

With the body and muscles warmed up and the pulse rate raised, it's time to move on to the aerobic component of our work-out in which we aim to improve heart and lung efficiency. But don't forget, you need to build up your aerobic exercising gradually. If you are a beginner, try doing four minutes. Better still, though, when you're at an intermediate level, is 12 minutes. Only then will you be gaining the enhanced benefit of working out. Your ultimate aim should be to go for the full 20-minute work-out for maximum benefit. But do take it gradually.

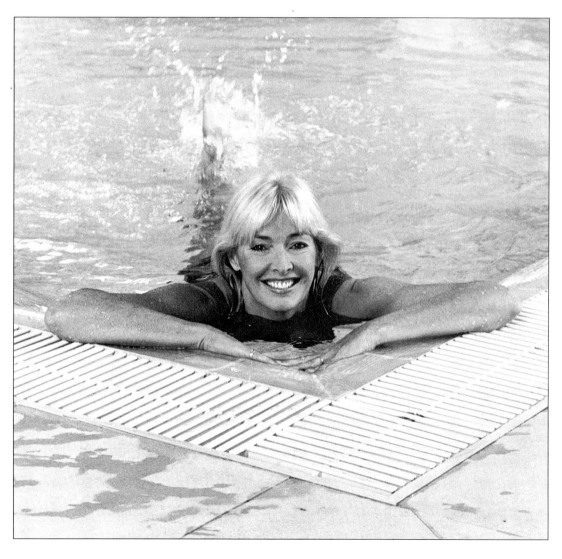

These exercises concentrate on the cardiovascular system (heart and lungs) and build up stamina. The pace should be gradually increased in order to make the body work harder and bring maximum benefit to the heart and lungs. This section will raise your pulse rate still higher and make you puff a bit. Remember to breathe deeply to give your muscles the oxygen they need to do their work. Work hard but don't get exhausted. Practice will make perfect, I promise. And when you're really into the swing of things, you should do these exercises at least three times a week to maintain a strong heart and lungs and build stamina.

But don't overdo it. Remember, aerobics means working with air. If we work too hard when we're stressed we work anaerobically (without air) and that will defeat the object of the exercise.

Don't forget that during an aerobic work-out, fat is attacked to provide energy for the muscles' activity and calories are used up. For a minimum of four minutes to help you burn off excess fat, build up your stamina and improve your heart and lung efficiency, put on some lively, motivating music and move.

Make a start by just walking on the spot. Lift your feet up and roll through the ball of your foot, and keep breathing easily. Use your arms to increase the intensity and keep going for one minute.

Now march forward for a count of four, swinging your arms. March on the spot for a count of four and then take four steps back. Turn to your left and repeat – marching forward for a count of four, and marching on the spot for a count of four. Move in this pattern, marching and turning, for one minute. You should start to feel warm and breathe more deeply.

Keep the music playing, and unless you are unsteady on your feet find a stair and simply step up and back down off it for another minute. Change your lead leg halfway through. Place your whole foot on the step for balance,

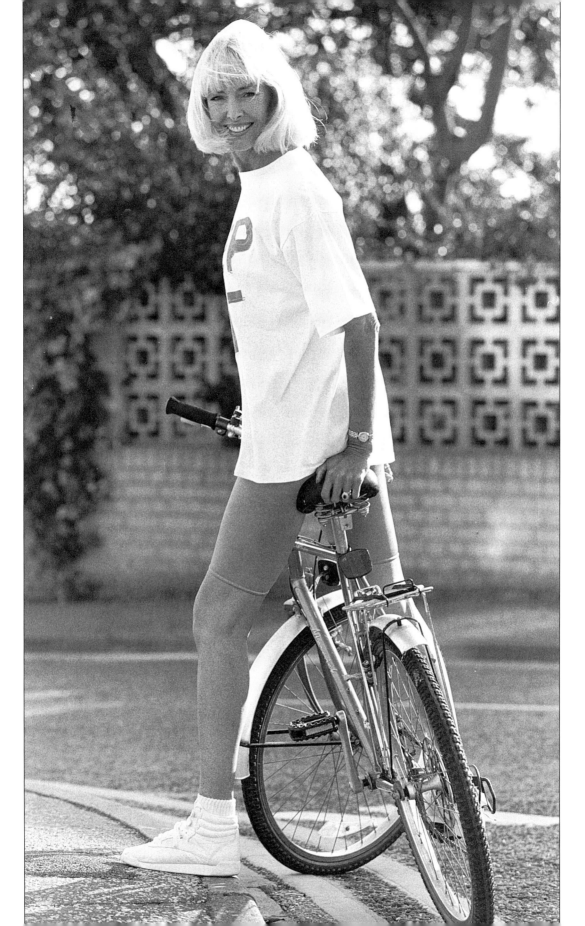

keep upright, remember your posture (tum in, bottom under), and keep your knees soft. You may be puffing a bit, so make sure you breathe easily. You should be able to speak. If you can't, and you feel exhausted, slow down gradually by just walking on the spot, and try again tomorrow. Now you are ready to pick and mix from the M.S.E. selection of exercises to strengthen your muscles. The rest of you, back to where you started, walking on the spot, but now simply step one foot out to the side and bring the other foot over to touch it. Repeat to the alternate side, transferring your weight from one foot to the other. Continue to 'step and touch', add some claps and enjoy the rhythm for another minute.

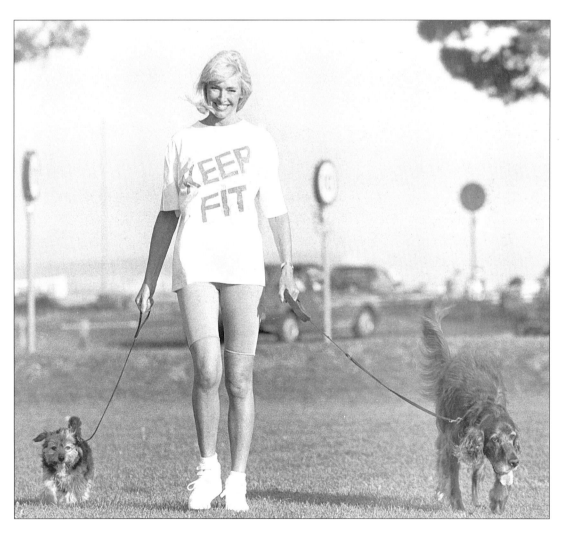

You need to build up your aerobic work, so that eventually you can do the full 20 recommended minutes. You could repeat these low impact movements, or you could put on an exercise video or audio tape. (*Ease Into Fitness* is available on Polygram video.)

Alternatively you could mix this section with another form of aerobic exercise in your own home. Maybe you have an exercise bike or a rowing machine, or a simple skipping rope is excellent aerobic exercise, but only for those of you who are more fit. A brisk walk in the fresh air is very beneficial. So too are bicycling and swimming. Both these exercises, apart from being very enjoyable, have the added advantage of supporting the bodyweight whilst you exercise – especially helpful if you have joint problems. Walks that take you up and down over varying gradients are particularly beneficial.

Any exercise to music should be fun, rhythmic and motivating, whether it's disco-dancing, ballroom dancing or a choreographed exercise routine. Whatever you do, keep your movements safe. Bring your heels down when you land to ensure that the movement is low impact. In high impact aerobics, the feet leave the ground and unless you are very fit, can result in injury.

So, pick and mix according to your mood, and gradually ease into fitness by achieving 20 minutes' aerobic work three times a week. But a word of warning: whatever activity you choose to do, don't stop suddenly. Bring the intensity of your movements down and gradually return your body to its pre-aerobic state. Your breathing should be normal by the end of your aerobic work. If not, just walk around until you feel completely relaxed. If you don't you may feel dizzy.

If, like me, you enjoy gardening, you can consider it as part of your exercise routine. All the bending and stretching will help keep you both strong and supple. But it will only count as 'aerobic' if you do vigorous, rhythmic movements, such as mowing the lawn with a push mower, sweep-

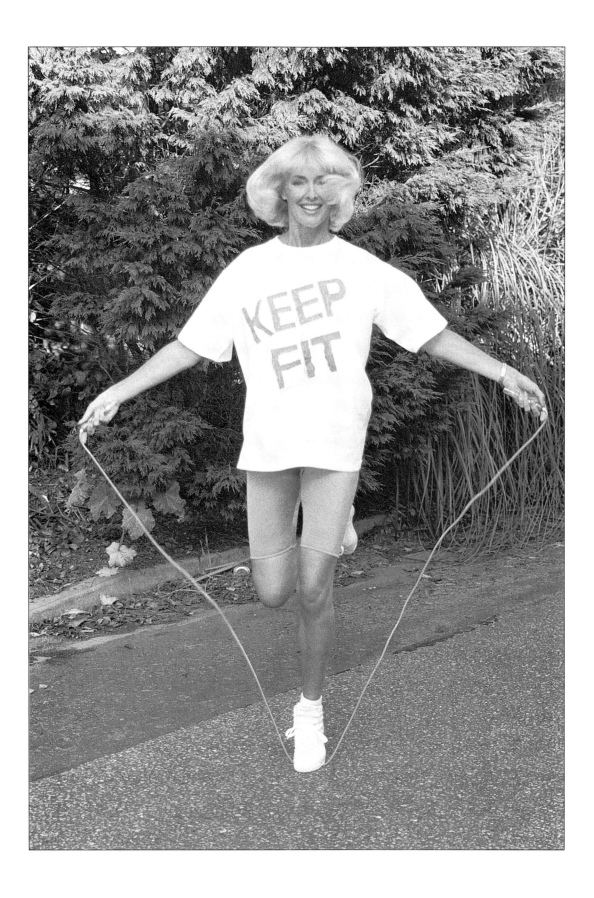

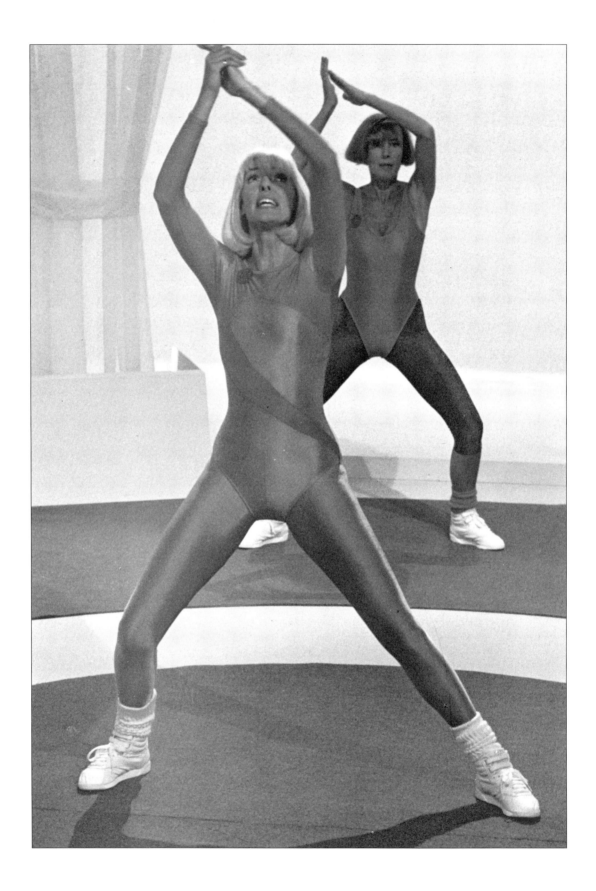

ing the paths or digging over the vegetable plot for a continuous 20 minutes. Just kneeling, doing the weeding, doesn't count!

Find an aerobic exercise that is fun to do. Maybe running or jogging – even jogging on the spot will do – and if you swim, then really swim laps for 20 minutes or make up your own dance routines. Whatever activity you choose, the bigger you make the movements, the greater the intensity. The more you give it, the more you will get from it.

After your Fat Attack of four minutes, 12 minutes or the full 20 minutes, you can move on to your choice from the M.S.E (Muscular Strength and Endurance) section. Or, if you wish, you can go immediately to the Relax/Stretch section. Whatever you choose to do, don't forget that it is essential to 'come down', and you must complete the Relax/Stretch section in full.

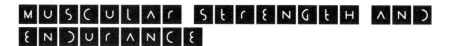

MUSCULAR STRENGTH AND ENDURANCE

This section will improve the tone of your muscles and shape up your body. Strong muscles will not only benefit your posture, they will also help you perform everyday tasks with ease and give you reserves of strength to tackle hobbies, sports and so on.

Each set of exercises concentrates on a particular 'problem area' which I know will worry most of us:

Tums

Bums

Thighs

Chest and Arms

Pick and mix according to your own particular needs. And if you have any physical disability, look out for the alternative positions which are equally beneficial in developing and maintaining stronger muscles.

The exercise should be done slowly and carefully with attention paid to correct positioning of the body. Do them at first in single time. Later on you can do them in double time to increase the intensity. In many cases, hand or leg weights can be added to further increase the intensity.

You should start these exercise gradually with four repetitions of each movement and build up to eight or more, again depending on your own individual goal.

22a *Pelvic 'Flaws'*

First a simple exercises to strengthen the pelvic floor – a sling of internal muscles which support the back passage, womb and bladder. No movement is visible when we perform this exercise.

Lie on your back, knees bent, feet apart, flat on the floor.

1. Tighten the muscles in the back passage.

2. Tighten the vagina.

3. Tighten the front passage (as if you are trying to stop spending a penny).

Slowly pull up all the muscles together as tight as you can and hold for a count of four. Relax.

Practise, and when you know what to do, close your eyes. It helps you concentrate on doing it correctly.

Do this uplifting exercise to tone the pelvic floor (or flaws as is often the case), whenever you think of it – lying in bed, in the bath, sitting watching TV or in the car, or you can even do it while you are just standing around. It is particularly beneficial after childbirth and for when we get older, as it helps to avoid gynaecological and incontinence problems. It will also improve our posture and help prevent backache.

22b *The Pelvic Tilt*

Lie in the same position. Pull in your abdominal muscles and tighten your bottom. Push your lower back down on to the floor. This will tilt your pelvis up and forward and get rid of the arch in your back.

You should hold this position throughout all the abdominal exercises and breathe in when you relax and out on effort.

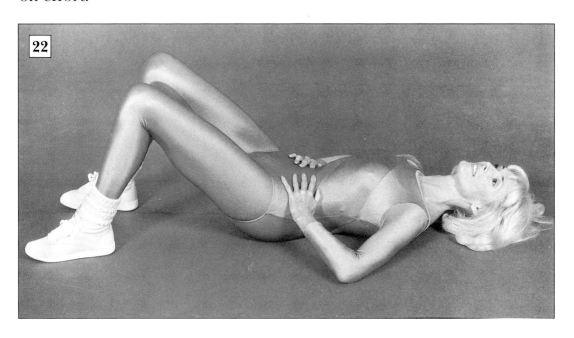

22

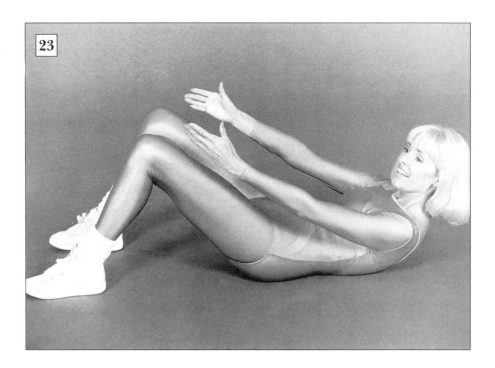

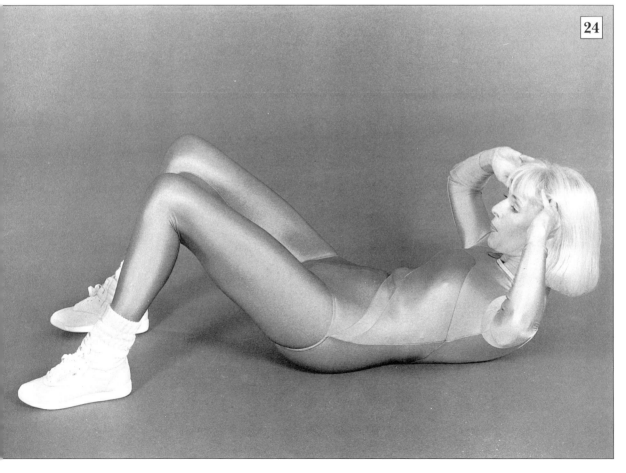

23 *To Strengthen the Central Abdominal Muscles*

Lie back on the floor (rest your head on a small cushion if it's more comfortable). Bend your knees and keep your feet flat on the floor. Reach your arms forward and place your hands on your thighs. Pull your tummy in, push your back down and tilt your pelvis. Breathe out and lift your head and shoulders and slide your hands up your thighs. Breathe in as you slowly relax back down.

To increase the intensity, cross your arms over your chest.

24

From the same position you can increase the intensity still further by placing your fingertips to your temples and keeping your elbows out to the sides. Remember your pelvic tilt, breathe out and lift your head and shoulders up. Keep your elbows back and don't jerk your head forward. Keep it steady and look through your legs as you come up. Relax down as your breathe in.

25 *To Strengthen the Crisscross Abdominal Muscles*

Lying in the same position, place one elbow on the floor, fingers to temple. 'Pelvic tilt' and breathe out. Lift your head and shoulders up and reach and touch the outside of your opposite knee with your outstretched hand. Breathe in and relax back down.

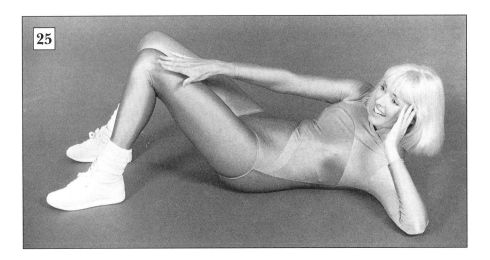

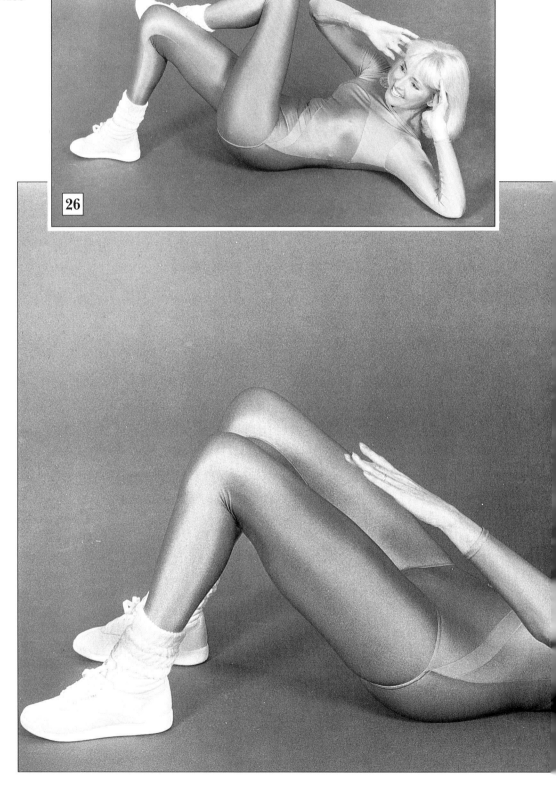

26

26 *To Strengthen the Crisscross Abdominal Muscles*
Lying in the same position, bend one elbow and place it on the floor out to the side. Place the fingertips of your other arm to your temples, and cross the knee on the same side over your other knee. Keep your elbow on the floor, tilt your pelvis, breathe out and lift your other arm up (raising head and shoulders), and reach across to touch the outside of your bent knee. Breathe in and relax back down.

Change legs and repeat.

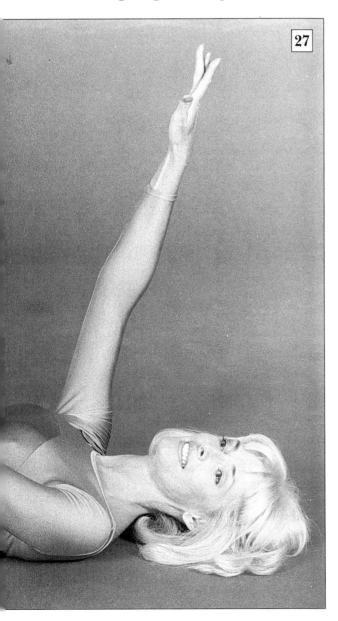

27 *Abdominal Rest*
You must always give your abdominal muscles a rest between each set of exercises. Lie on your back, knees bent and back pressed into the floor. Slowly sweep alternate arms up past your ears and back over your head. Bring them back up again past your ears and down. Repeat 4 times slowly.

If you are a beginner aim to do 3 sets of 8 repetitions of both the central and crisscross abdominal exercises. As your technique improves, increase the number of repetitions and eventually move on to the harder position.

These exercises are safe but strong, so don't do too much, too soon and overstrain your muscles.

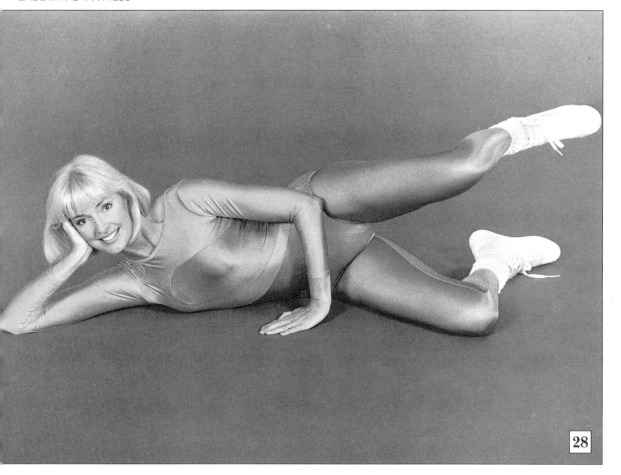

28

28 *To Work the Abductor (Outer Thigh Muscles)*
Lie on your side, bend your knees and bring them forward.
Bend your elbow and rest your head in one hand. Place the
other hand in front of your body to support it. Don't
roll backwards or forwards. Pull in your tummy and tighten
your bottom. Lift your bent upper leg up (not too high),
keep your foot lower than the knee and don't drop your hip
back. Take the leg up and lower it back down with control,
flexing your foot and leading with your heel. (Bent leg is a
half lever.)

29

If you find the previous exercise too easy, lie as before but keep your lower leg bent back but with your thigh in line with your upper body. Straighten your upper leg (full lever). This increases the intensity. You could add leg weights to increase the intensity still further. Remember to keep the tum and bum tight throughout the exercise.

Roll over and repeat the exercise with the other leg, taking care not to roll backwards or forwards while doing it.

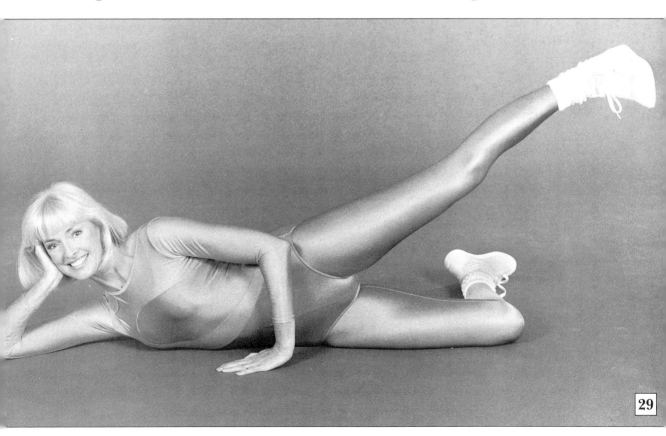

29

30 *To Work the abductors (Inner Thigh Muscles)*

From your choice of lying position (28 or 29), take your top leg over and place your knee down comfortably in front of you for support. Straighten out your lower leg and take it back so that it is in line with your upper body. Flex your foot and, leading with your heel, lift and lower your leg with small controlled movements. Feel the inner thigh muscles working.

Roll over and repeat exercises on the other side.

If you cannot get on to the floor or wish to take advantage of exercising anywhere, any time, try the same two exercises but standing sideways against a wall or a chair for support.

Remember your posture and with your hand on your hip, take your outside leg out and up to the side, leading with

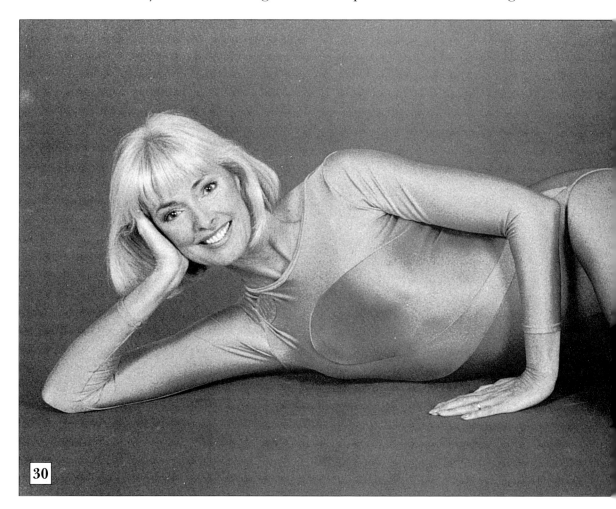

30

the heel and keeping the supporting knee soft. Control the movement up and down and work the outside thigh.

To work the inside thigh, lead with your heel and simply take the same leg across in front of your body with small controlled movements.

31 *For Backs of Thighs (not illustrated)*
Now roll onto your tummy, with your head on your hands. Slowly bend your knee and bring one foot up behind you to touch your bottom (or as near as comfortable). Control the movement up and down, and feel the back of your thigh working. Repeat 4 times. Change legs, and work the other side.

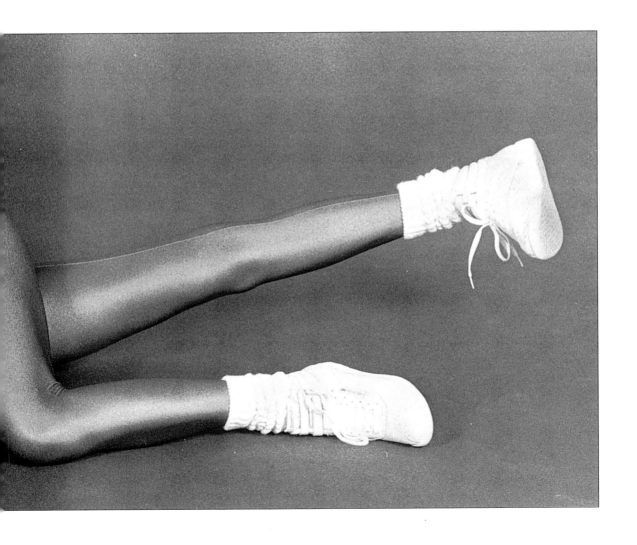

32 *For Front of Thighs*
Sit back comfortably, resting on your elbows, knees bent,
and feet flat on the floor. Straighten one leg out, flex the
foot and lift your leg up to the level of your other knee.
Control the movement both up and down. Pull in your
tummy and don't arch your back. Change legs and repeat.

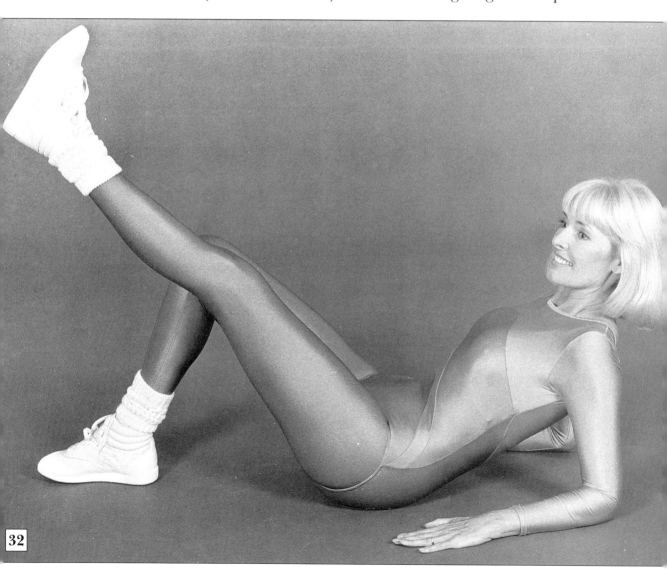

32

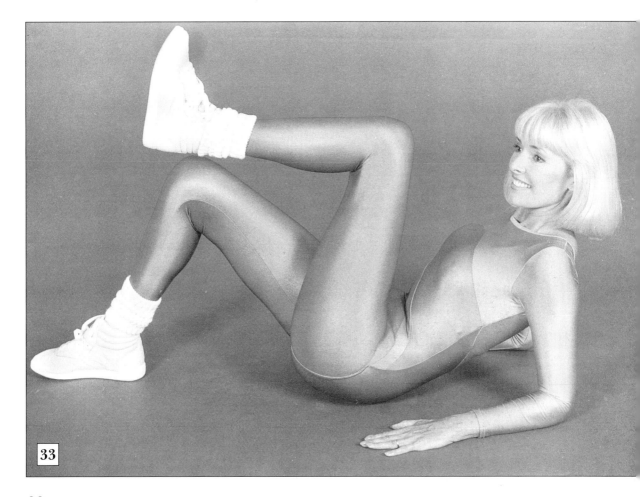

33

From the same position bring one knee back into your chest, straighten and 'push' it out in front, then lift and lower with control. Repeat the in/out, out/up, up/down movement rhythmically. Repeat with the other leg.

Begin with 3 sets of 8 repetitions of each exercise but alternate them for any specific muscle. By adding leg weights to the last three exercises, you will increase the intensity. As you gain strength, build up the number of repetitions to suit your individual needs.

MSE – BUMS

34 *To Tighten Bottom Muscles*

Stand behind a chair and hold on for support. Straighten one leg back and rest your toes on the floor. Pull your tummy in and keep the bottom tight. Slightly incline your upper body and keep your hips facing forward. Slowly raise and lower your straight leg up behind you with little lifts and feel the bottom muscles working. Change legs and repeat.

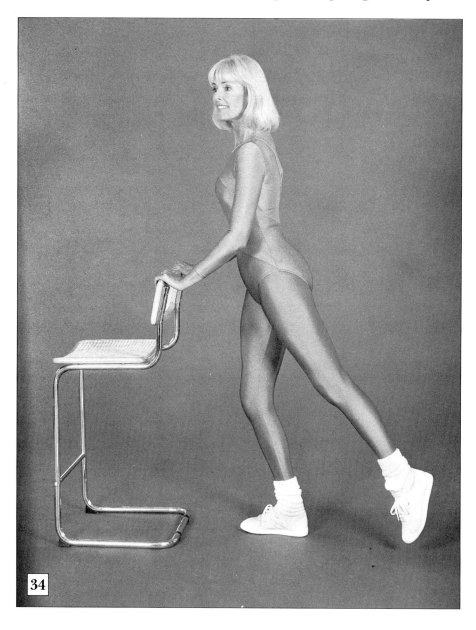

35 *To Tone Your Thighs and Tighten Your Bottom*

Stand behind the chair, legs wider apart and toes facing out diagonally. Bend your knees out over your toes and with your back straight and tummy and bottom tight, lower down as far as comfortable and up again with control. Keep your heels down.

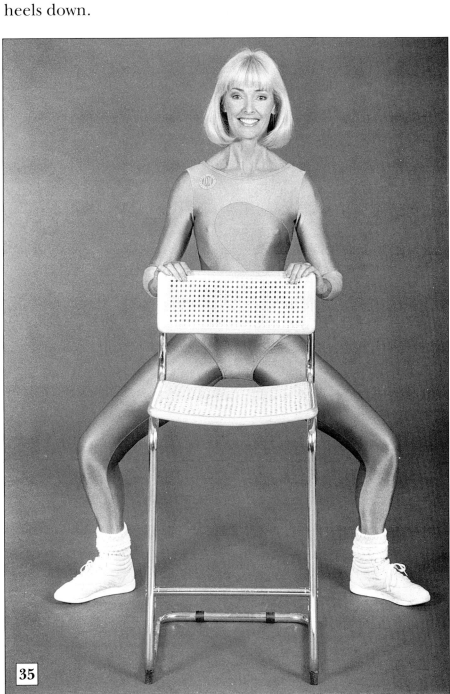

35

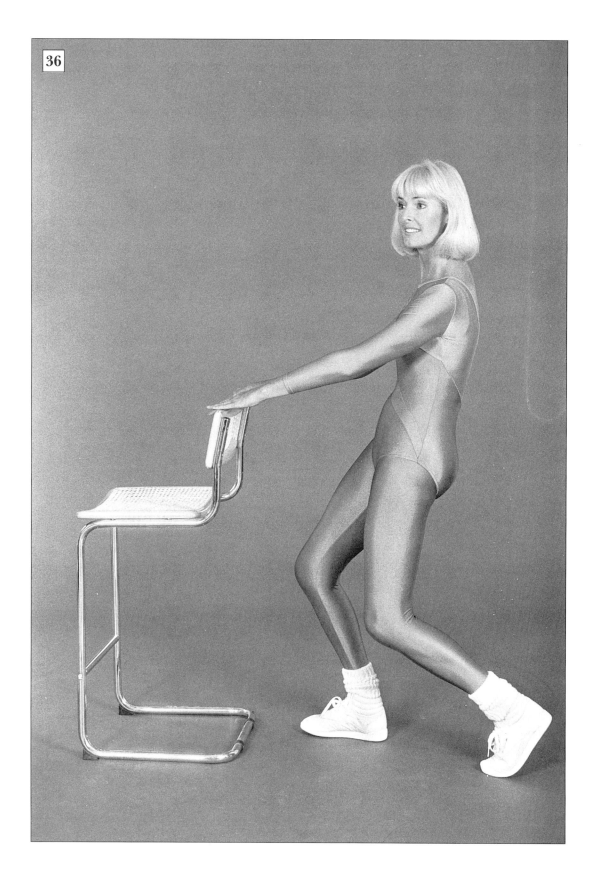

36

36 *To Tighten Bottom Muscles*

Stand nearer to the back of the chair and hold onto it for support. Place one foot, hip width apart, a little behind the other. Bend both your knees, tilt your pelvis forward, and keep your bottom tight. Keep your back straight and go down as if you were sitting back on a stool. Don't bend your front knee more than 90 degrees. Tighten your bottom muscles and raise your body back up. Continue the up and down movement rhythmically with control.

37

Kneel on the floor, bend your elbows and place them under your shoulders, fingers facing forward and inwards. Lift one leg back and up, bending the knee at 90 degrees and keeping the thigh parallel with the floor, (half lever). Lift and lower with a small movement, keeping both hips facing down and knee bent. Feel the bottom muscles working, but don't let your hip raise up or out to the side. Control both the up and down movement. Repeat for the other leg.

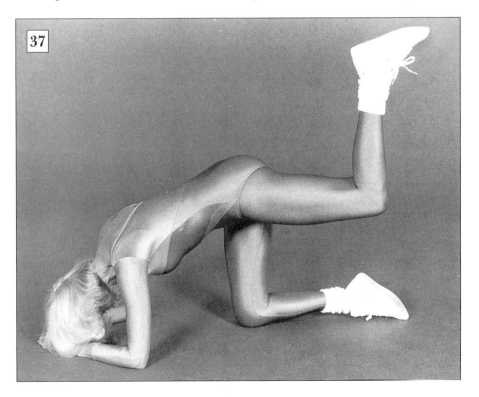

38 *To Tighten Bottom Muscles*

As before, but increase the intensity by working with a straight leg (full lever), and further increase the intensity by using leg weights. It is important to pull up the tummy muscles throughout these exercises to prevent the body sagging.

If this position is uncomfortable, go down still further and place your head on your hands on the floor.

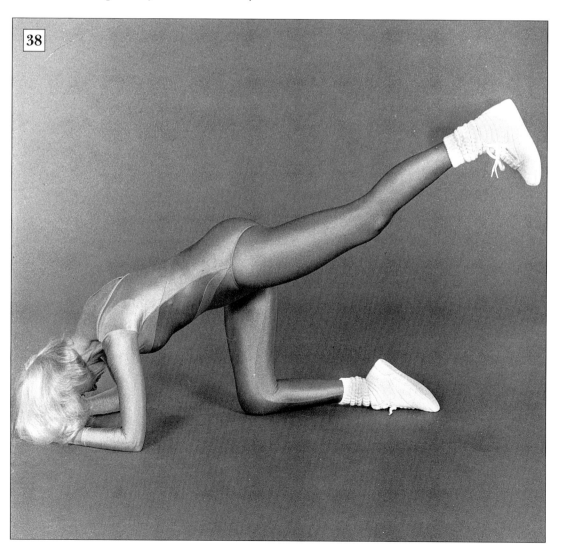

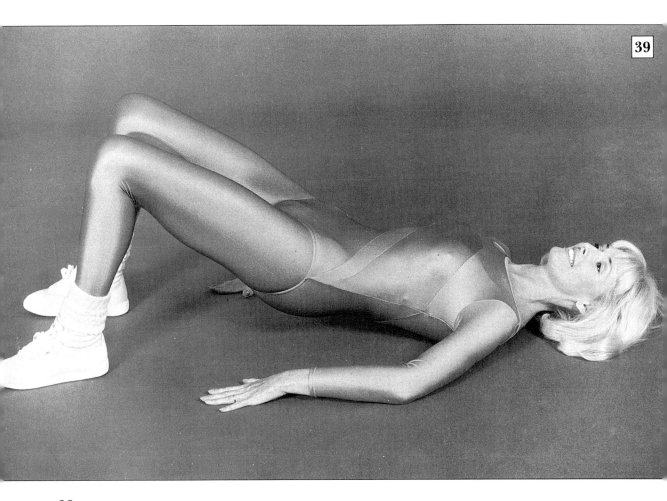

39

This fun exercise adds variety and helps firm the thighs as well as the bottom. Lie on your back, knees bent, feet together flat on the floor. Simply clench and lift up your bottom, squeezing your thigh, knees and ankles together (don't lift too high, and keep your shoulders on the floor).

Begin all these exercises with 3 sets of 8 repetitions, and build up to suit your individual requirements.

MSE – ARMS AND CHEST

You can sit or stand for these exercises.

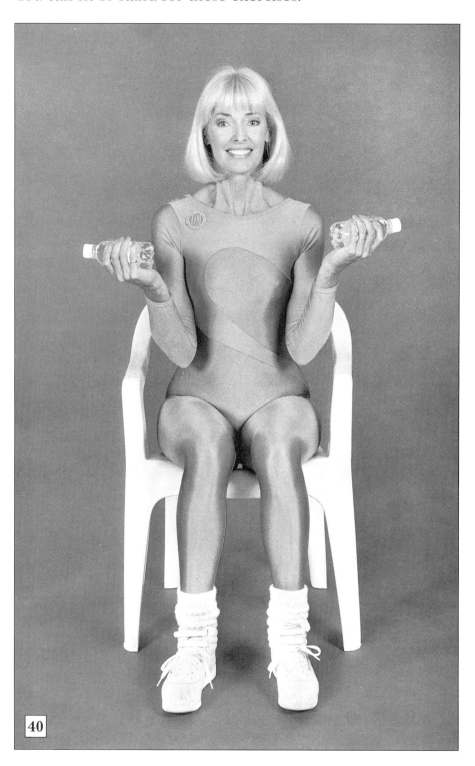

40

40 *To Strengthen and Shape Front Upper Arm Muscle (Biceps)*

Sit upright in a chair with your feet flat on the floor and knees at right angles. Remember your posture. Tuck your elbows into your waist and simply imagine you're lifting a weight. Raise your lower arm up, fists to shoulder, and back down. To add intensity, use hand weights or plastic drinks bottles filled with water or sand.

41 *For the Triceps (Back Upper Arm)*

Make a fist or use weights. Take your upper arms back behind you and keep them completely still. Push your lower arm out behind you, taking care not to lock the elbow. Keep your upper arm steady as you bend your elbow and bring your fist back up to your shoulder. Feel the back of your upper arm working. Incline your upper body forward slightly and pull in your stomach muscles to maintain a good position.

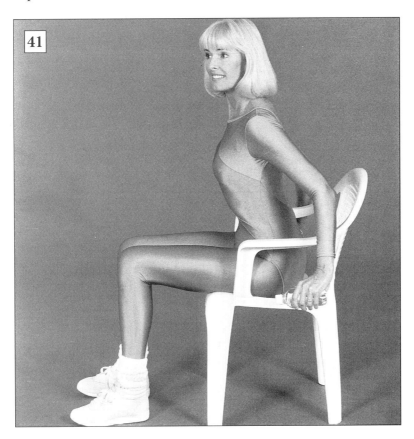

42 *For the Shoulder, Middle Back and Side Muscles*
Take your arms out wide to the sides, and keeping them out straight, lift them up to shoulder level only and down again with a slow controlled movement. Keep your shoulders down and relaxed, and don't lock your elbows. Use weights to add intensity.

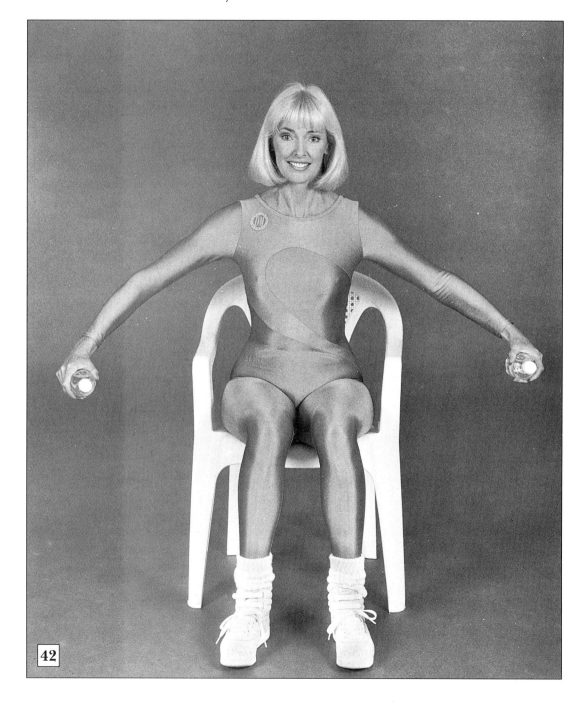

42

43

From a seated position (remembering your posture), take your fists to your shoulders. Simply raise and lower your arms above your head, controlling both the up and down movements and keeping your shoulders relaxed. Use weights to add intensity.

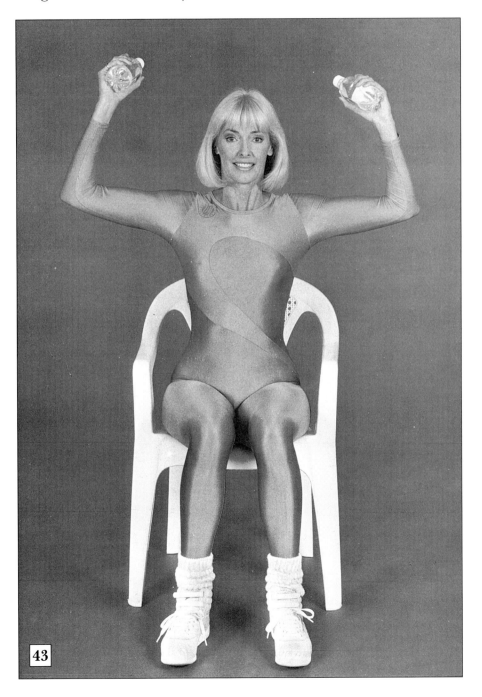

43

44 *To Work the Triceps (Back of Your Upper Arm)*
Sit down on the floor with your hands back under your shoulders for support, fingers facing forward. Pull in your tummy, press your back down and keeping your upper body in a straight line, lower backwards, bending only your elbows. Work the back of your arms and raise your body back up with controlled movements. To add to the intensity of this exercise, lift your bottom up off the floor. Remember to breathe out on effort and in as you relax back down.

45 *To Work the Pectorals (Chest Muscles)*
Kneel and place your hands on the floor a little more than shoulder width apart, fingers facing forward and inward. Pull up the tummy and keep your back and head in a straight line. Bend the elbows out and lower your upper body down to touch your forehead to the floor (or as far as is comfortable). Straighten your elbows and come back up with control. Don't overstrain. And remember to breathe correctly.

46
To add to the intensity, take your knees back further and cross your ankles if you find this more comfortable. You can do this exercise with straight legs if you are very strong. Continue to lift and lower, pulling up the abdominal muscles, keeping a straight back and bending your elbows only, not your body Alternatively, if you have difficulty getting down to the floor, you can easily do this exercise standing up against a wall. Stand a foot or so away, place your hands on the wall at shoulder level, bend your elbows out and lower your upper body into the wall. Keep your heels down and don't let your body sag in the middle.

Start the seated exercises with 3 sets of 8 repetitions. The floor exercises are tough. Start by doing 2 sets of 4 repetitions of each exercise and build up as you gain strength. Listen to your body and build up gradually. Stop if it hurts.

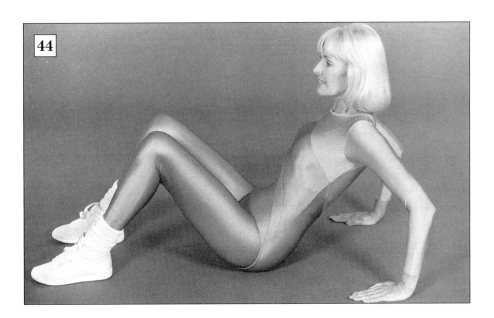

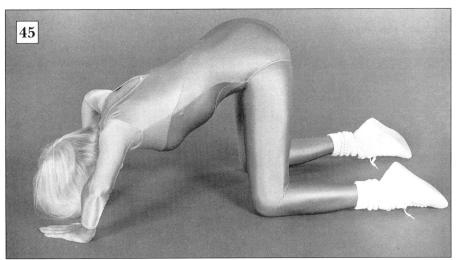

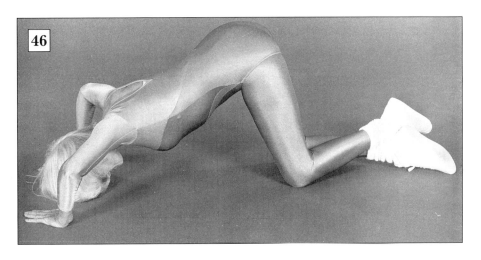

MSE – BACKS

These exercises will strengthen your back, but take care. If you have a bad back, consult your doctor before doing these or any exercises.

47

Lie out on your tummy with your head on the floor. Take your hands behind your back and either clasp them together or rest them on your bottom. Breathe out and raise up your chest, shoulders and head. Keep your head in a

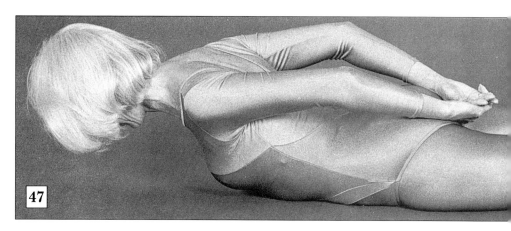

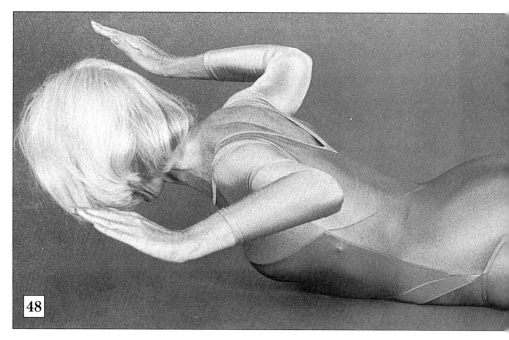

straight line with your body and look down. Breathe in and lower back down. Repeat this movement slowly and carefully 4 times.

48 *To Help 'Round Shoulders'*

Lie out on your tummy with your nose to the floor. Take your arms out to the sides, bend your elbows (90 degrees), and keep your arms out to the front but higher than shoulder level. Pull your shoulders back together, breathe out and slowly lift your arms and hands off the ground, raising your head and shoulders back and up, like a bird in

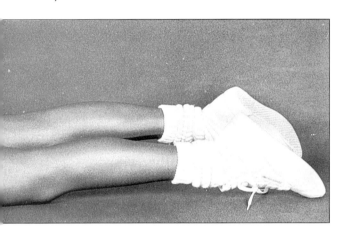

flight. If you find this position uncomfortable, keep your head down on the floor and only work with your arms. Start with 4 repetitions and build up as you gain strength.

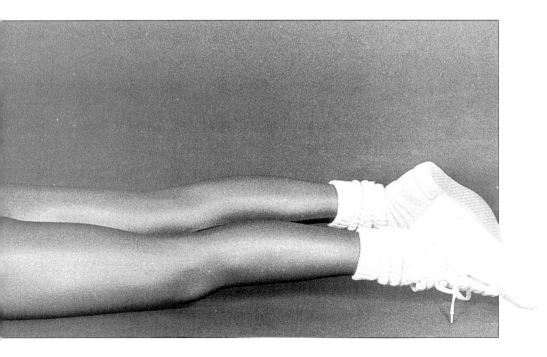

RELAX / STRETCH

It is essential to come down and relax the body after working it hard. Muscles which are warm can be returned to their pre-exercise state and certain muscles such as the hamstrings at the back of the thighs which tighten from wearing high heels or too much sitting can be stretched out a little further. This will improve flexibility, suppleness and general mobility (more and more essential as we get older!)

You should do this complete section after your work-out, whatever you've chosen to pick and mix beforehand.

49 *Whole Body Stretch*

Lie on your back on the floor with your legs comfortably apart and your arms at your sides. Close your eyes and keep breathing deeply into your tummy. Slowly sweep one arm out along the floor and up behind your head. Repeat with the other arm.

Stretch out one arm, taking the stretch right through to your fingertips. Now stretch the other arm. Stretch out your shoulders, your chest, your back.

Lengthen and stretch one leg and the other and stretch out the toes. Lengthen and stretch out your entire body and hold for 10 seconds (but don't stop breathing). Release and relax and let go. Let your legs and feet flop out to the side and let your mind and body float.

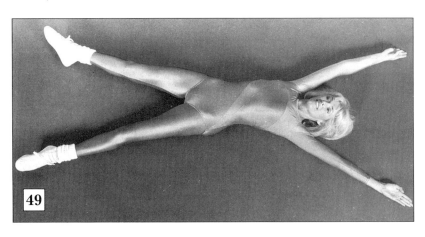

49

50 *Hamstring Stretch (Back of Thigh)*

Lie on your back with the knees bent and feet flat on the floor. Holding behind the thigh, bring one knee up to your chest. Take your hand behind your calf and extend your leg. You don't need to straighten it. Feel the stretch in your hamstring. Hold for 8-10 seconds. You can develop this stretch further by gently easing your thigh closer to your chest and holding for a further 10 seconds. Repeat with the other leg.

This stretch is an important one. Hamstring muscles tighten from too much sitting and from wearing high-heeled shoes.

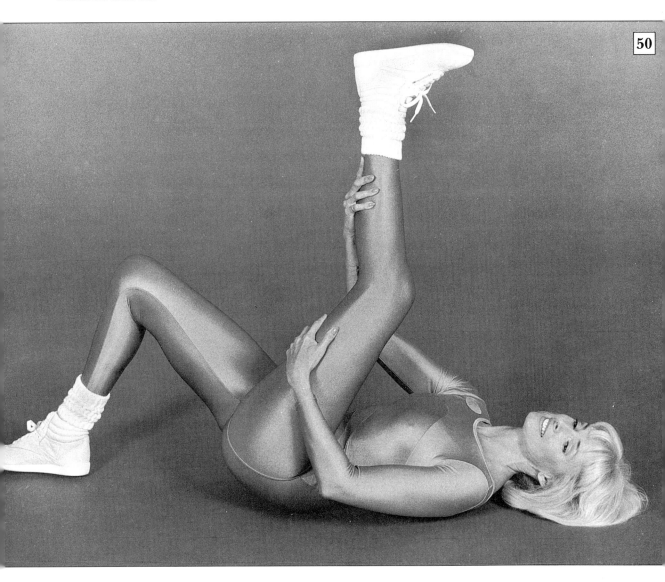

50

51 *Obliques (Across the Tummy)*

Lie on your back and extend your arms out to the sides, with your palms facing down. Keep your feet in contact with the floor and twist only from your waist. Take your knees

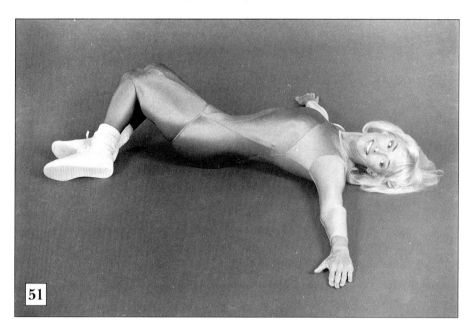

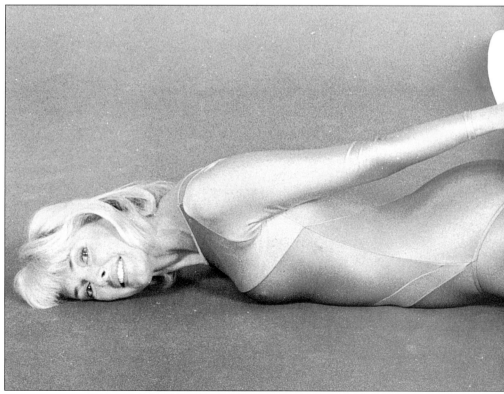

over to one side of your body to touch the floor (or as far as comfortable). Look over to your opposite hand, hold and feel the stretch across your body for 10 seconds. Repeat to the other side and always keep your shoulders down on the floor.

52 *Quadriceps Stretch (Front Thigh)*
Roll over on to your tummy and keep your head and shoulders down on the floor. Reach behind you, bend one knee and grasp your ankle (not your toes) and gently ease your foot towards your bottom, or as far as comfortable, and feel the stretch in the front thigh. Hold for 10 seconds. If you find this difficult, hold on to your sock or use a towel around your ankle to help. Repeat with the other leg. Develop this stretch by holding for a further 10 seconds.

This stretch can be performed standing by a support if you have trouble getting down.

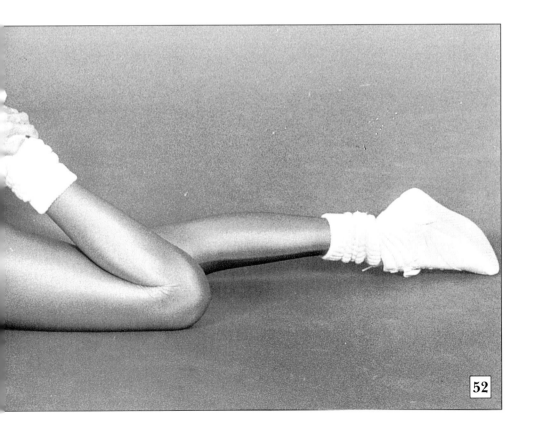

53 *Abdominal Stretch (Tummy)*

Lie straight out on your tummy and place your elbows under your shoulders, fingers facing forward and inward. Rest on your elbows and push your head, chest and shoulders up and back, but keep your hips in contact with the floor. Look up and hold the stretch for 10 seconds.

54 *Shoulder Stretch*

Come up on to your knees and stick your bottom up in the air. Stretch your arms out in front and slide them forward carefully, lowering your chest to the floor as far as is comfortable. Feel the stretch across your shoulders and hold it for 10 seconds.

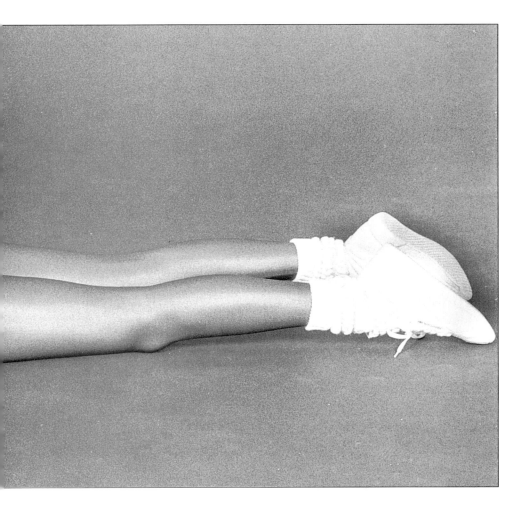

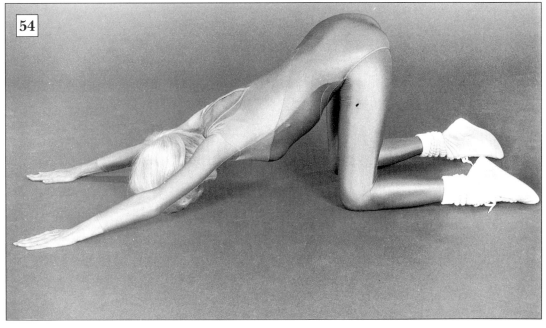

55 *Back Stretch*

Kneel up and place your hands under your shoulders, fingers facing forward. Drop your head down to look between your knees and at the same time pull up your tummy muscles, clench your buttocks (pelvic tilt again!) and round and stretch out your back. Hold for 10 seconds.

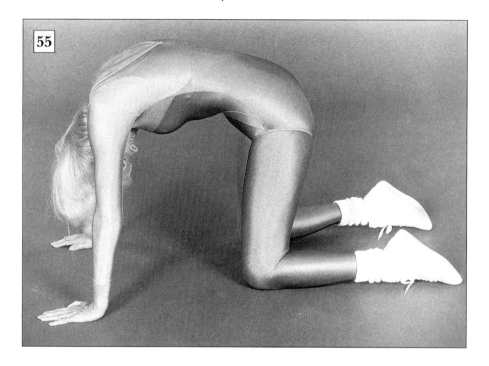

56

Relax your back down. An ideal opportunity to practise improving your pelvic 'flaws'!

57 *Bottom Stretch*

Sit with your legs outstretched, bend one knee and take your foot over the other leg and place it flat on the floor by the side of the straight knee. Take your opposite arm over and around the knee, placing your hand on your outer thigh. Place your other hand on the floor behind your bottom for support. Breathe in and sit up straight. Breathe out and twist your upper body and head around to look over your shoulder. Hold for 10 seconds and feel the stretch in your bottom. Repeat with the other leg.

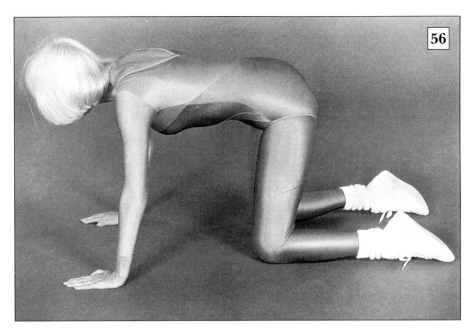

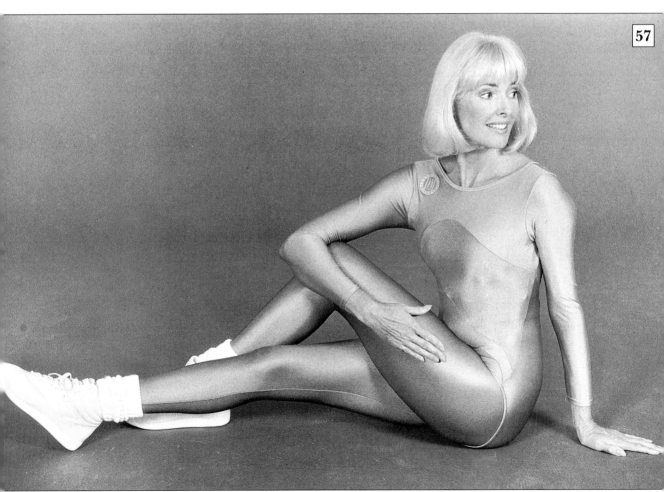

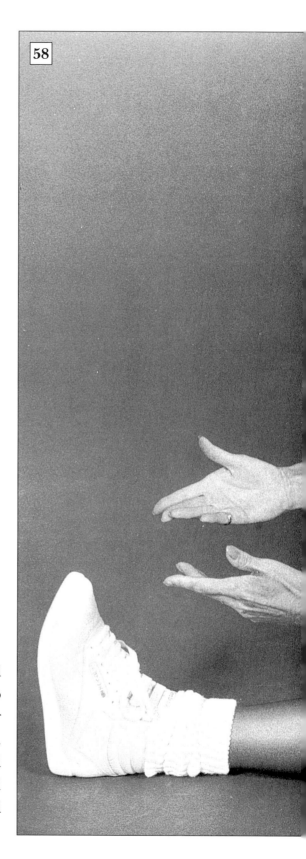

58 *Lower Back Stretch*

Sit with your legs outstretched. Bend
one leg and let the knee drop out to
the side and place the flat of your
foot by the side of your other knee.
Breathe in and sit up. Breathe out and
stretch both arms forward, and feel
the stretch in your lower back. Hold
for 10 seconds.

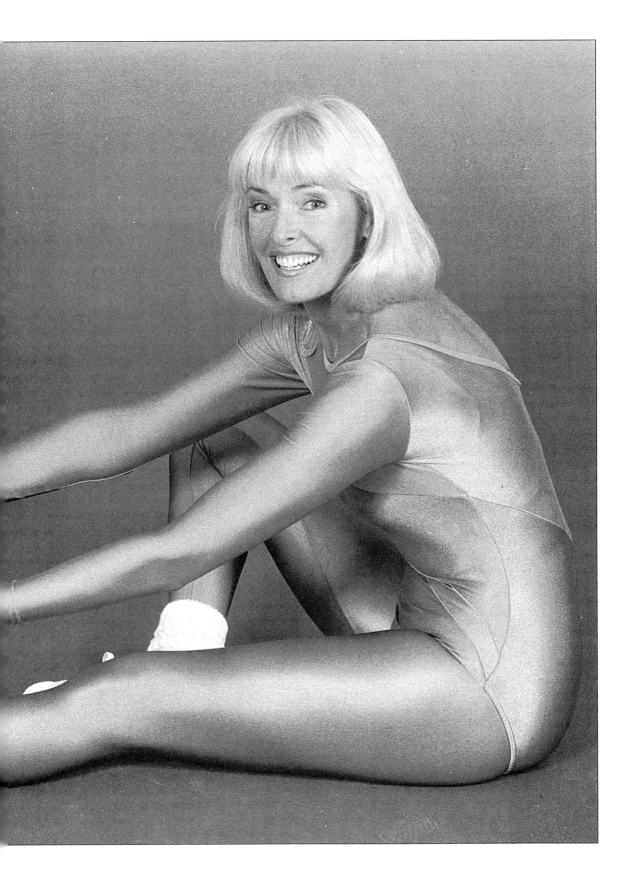

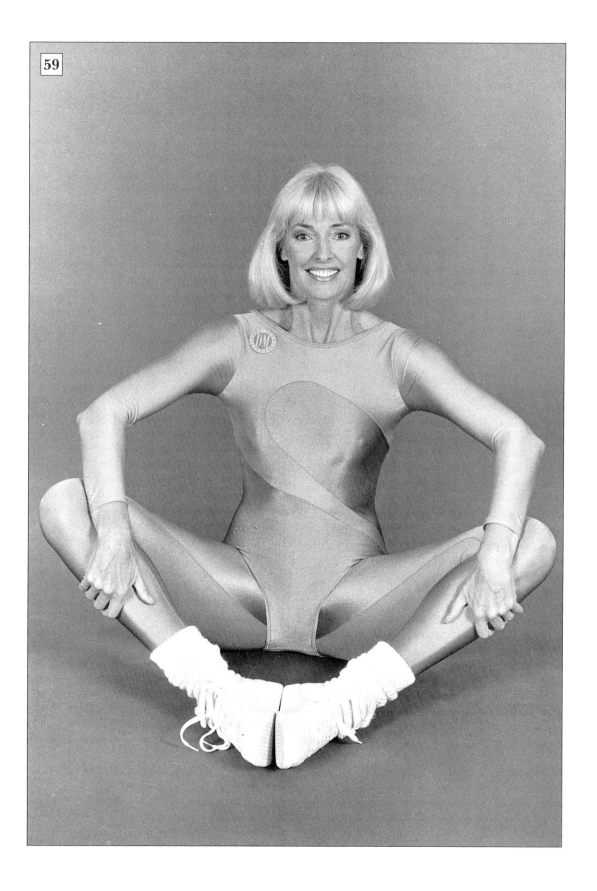

59 *Groin and Thigh Stretch*

Sit with the soles of your feet together and your knees out to the sides. Remember your posture. Pull your tummy in, bottom tight and sit up tall. Place your hands on your knees and gently push them down and feel the stretch in your groin and inner thighs. Hold for 10 seconds. Develop the stretch still further by holding for another 10 seconds.

60 *Back Stretch*

From the same positition as the previous stretch, or if you find it more comfortable straighten out one leg. Clasp your hands together in front of your chest and 'round out' your upper back (give someone an imaginary hug). Hold for 10 seconds.

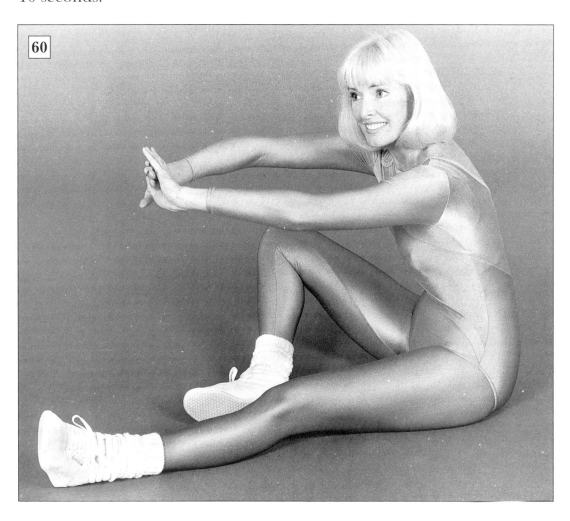

61 *Chest Stretch*

From the same position, take your arms behind your back, clasp your hands together, pull your shoulders back and stretch out your chest. Hold for 10 seconds, but don't arch your back.

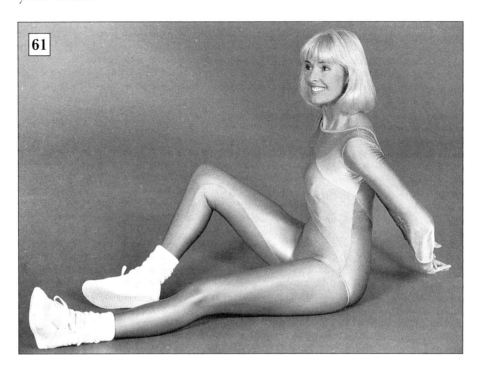

62 *Latissims Dorsi Stretch (Sides)*

Kneel up and stretch one leg straight out to the side, but keep your foot facing forward and flat on the floor. Raise your arm on the same side and reach up to take your body over. Use your other arm to support you, hand on the floor and keep your hips facing forward but don't bend forward or backward. Feel the beautiful stretch from your upper arm through the side of your body. Hold for 10 seconds.

Reverse and stretch the other side.

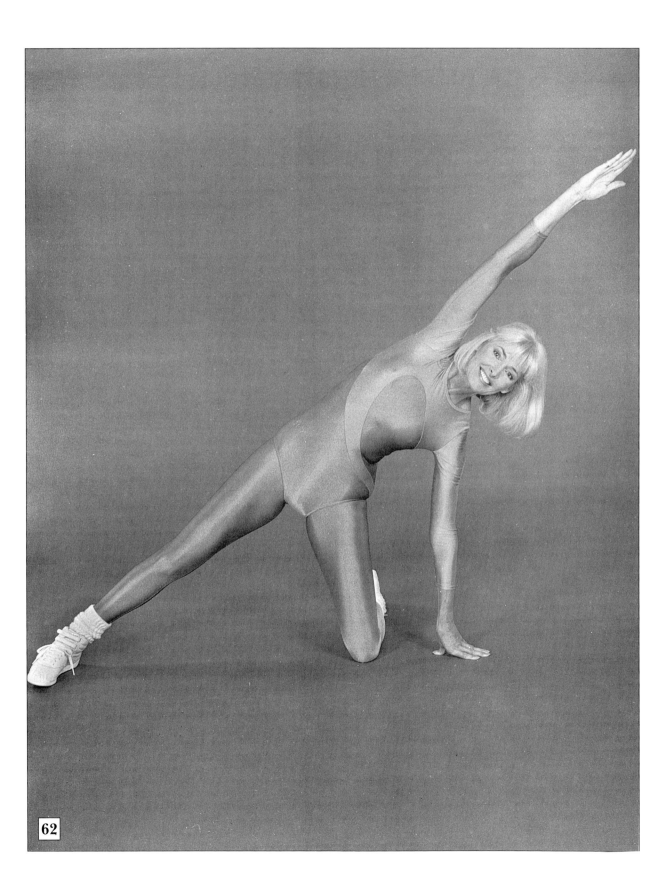

62

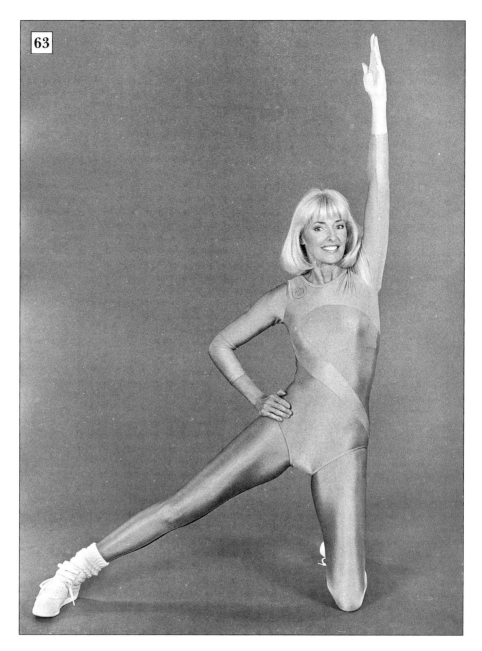

63 *Abductor Stretch (Inside Thigh)*

From the same position as 62, and keeping your leg out to the side, simply raise the other arm up or put your hand on your waist. Keep your hips facing forward and feel the stretch in the inside thigh. Hold for a further 5 seconds.

Reverse knees and stretch to the other side.

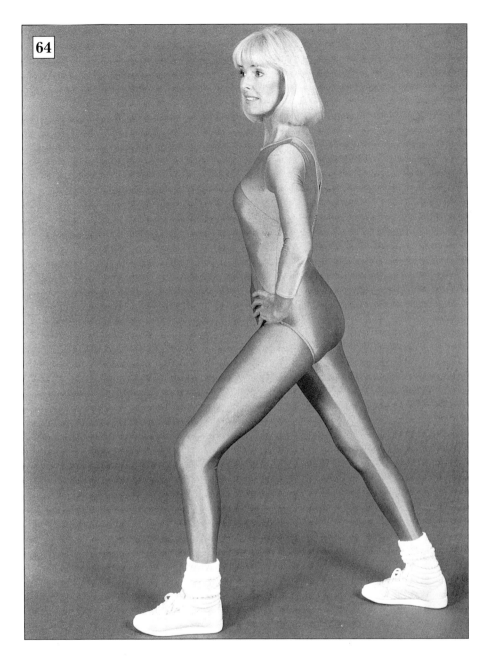

64 *Calf Stretch*
Stand with one foot, toes facing forward, and bend the knee. Take the other foot back behind you with the knee straight, place it hip width apart, toes facing forward and push your heel down. If need be, take the foot back still further until you feel the stretch in your calf. Remember your posture and keep your body upright. Hold for 10 seconds and then repeat for the other leg.

65 *For the Lower Calf*

Now bring your back foot forward and place it hip width apart just behind the front foot. Bend both knees but transfer the weight on to your back leg.

Keep your body upright, tummy pulled in, bottom tight and with the pelvis tilted forward. Both feet should be facing forward. Feel the stretch low down at the bottom of the calf and around the heel. Hold for 10 seconds.

66 *A Complete Body Stretch*

Stand with your legs wide apart and reach both hands high to the ceiling. Continue breathing deeply, lift up the rib cage, pull in your tummy, tighten your bottom and stretch throughout your body from your feet to your fingertips. Hold for 10 seconds.

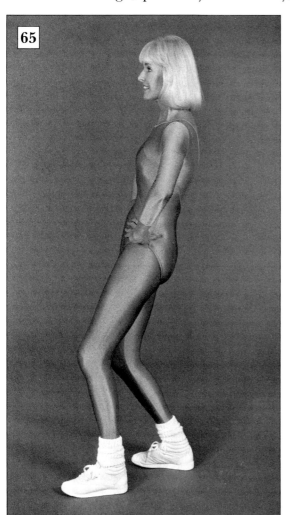

As you become more flexible, try holding some of the stretches a little longer to improve your suppleness.

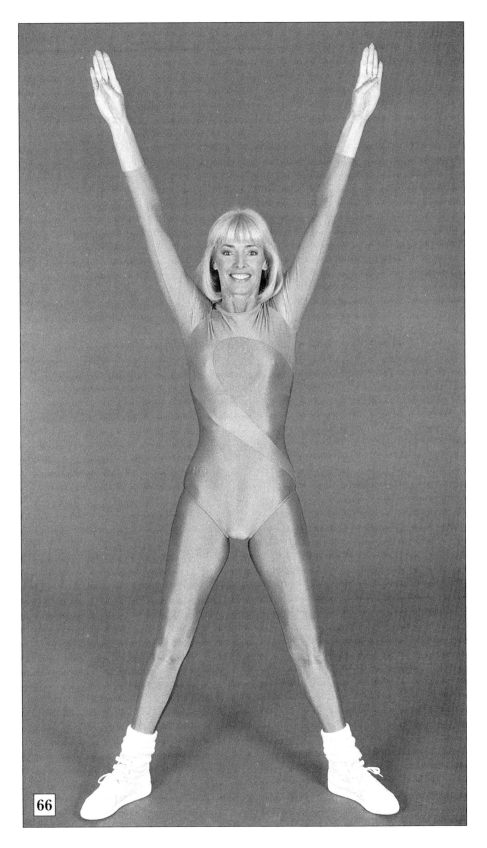

66

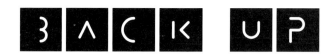

ack pain affects most of us at some time in our lives and accounts for a staggering figure of approximately 33 million working days lost in Britain every year.

We can avoid much of the trouble by checking out our posture and taking a little more care. Backache is often caused by strain, and more attention to how we sit, stand, lift and carry might avoid a lot of the problems.

Take a look at yourself in the mirror. Try to stand with your weight equally on both feet, tummy pulled in, bottom tucked under, with your shoulders back but down and relaxed. Keep your head up and try not to slouch.

During movement, exercise, lifting and carrying, keep your knees soft, not locked at the joint. When you need to bend down, bend the knees and do not move over and forward from the waist with your legs straight. Always bend your knees not your back. When you lift heavy objects make your legs do the work and also make certain you keep the weight held tightly into your body. Why not ask someone else to help you with really heavy objects? It's better to be safe than sorry and laid up in bed for weeks.

Learn the technique of the pelvic tilt (see p.73) and apply this when you're standing, walking, exercising, sitting or lying down. It's important that the abdominal (tummy) muscles should be strong and that they work in conjunction with the back muscles. This controls our posture and prevents bad backs.

If your job or your way of life involves a lot of sitting it's extremely important that you have your chair at the correct height. Don't settle for less than the correct seated position. Even a small cushion can raise you up or support your back. And a block of wood or telephone directory under your feet can make all the difference if your legs are short and don't touch the floor. Be certain that your bench or desk is at a comfortable height and that you are in near enough to it to avoid hunching forward. If you look at a screen all day check that you're not craning up or peering down. You should look straight into it to avoid strain. Crossing your legs will only encourage bad circulation and varicose veins. So sit with your feet flat on the floor or loosely crossed at he ankle. Try to keep your tummy pulled in at all times and press the small of your back into the chair. A slouch will only cause backache.

If your shoulders and neck and upper back do become stiff, try to do some of the mobility exercises from the Warm Up section of the exercise programme. Most of them can be done while you're still sitting but will help loosen your muscles and joints and relieve tension. Don't end up carrying the cares of the world on your shoulders!

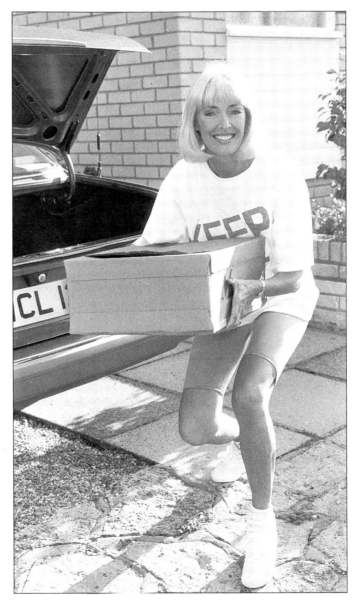

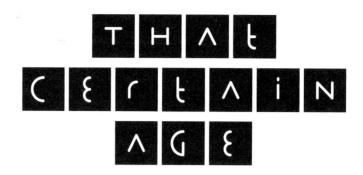

THAT CERTAIN AGE

The menopause is a natural part of every woman's life. Her periods come to an end and she is no longer able to bear children. In simple terms, apart from her ovaries ceasing to produce eggs, her body is also stopping the production of oestrogen and progesterone – the two female hormones that were responsible during puberty for turning her from a girl into a woman. The average age for the menopause is 50, but for some women it can be as early as 35 and for others as late as 60. For the vast majority of women the menopause also marks a new beginning in their lives.

Going through the menopause means different things to different women. About 25 per cent experience no problems at all. Fifty per cent find themselves mildly affected, and another 25 per cent experience severe problems such as hot flushes and sweating – symptoms that can last for a few months or in some cases a few years.

The hormonal changes that are going on in the body during this time can also cause drying and thinning of the vaginal wall and a loss of lubrication, causing discomfort during intercourse. And some women feel tired and listless and complain of backache, pains in their joints, drying of the skin and hair.

Besides coping with 'the change', there are often many other significant adjustments going on in a woman's life at this time. The children may have grown and flown. A husband may be having a mid-life crisis of his own – many do, you know. All in all it's not surprising that many women find themselves becoming irritable, unsure of themselves and the future, and flustered into forgetting things.

While many sail through the menopause, others who are not so lucky must decide whether or not to put up with the problems they experience, hoping they'll soon pass, or decide to seek help. Some doctors will nowadays offer support in the form of hormone replacement therapy (H.R.T.). Others may not be so keen.

If the menopause is allowed its natural progression, the periods become irregular and eventually stop. If you decide to take H.R.T., be prepared for a withdrawal bleed each month. If the thought of your periods continuing long-term daunts you, then H.R.T. is not for you. But for many women, it's a small price to pay for the disappearance of the sometimes severe and unpleasant symptoms of the menopause. Remember, what is good for one woman is not necessarily good for another, and if after taking suitable advice you do embark on H.R.T. you may find it takes some time to achieve the correct treatment and dosage for your own body.

Once on H.R.T. many women find that their aches, pains and skin problems improve, they feel better in themselves and find it easy to get back to 'normal'. The embarrassing daytime flushes which can be so distressing for some disappears, and they and their husbands or partners can experience a good night's sleep without her breaking out in a sweat and tossing and turning the whole night through.

Of course H.R.T. can only be given under medical supervision and some women may be advised that it is not suitable for them. It may also be prescribed for the menopause only or on a long-term basis. There is an increasing number of clinics with specialist advice on menopausal problems who have the most up-to-date expertise on its suitability in individual cases.

Before putting any woman on H.R.T. doctors will require a woman's complete medical history and give her a full

TOP TIP

Take advantage of screening programmes for cervical and breast cancer. Better to be safe than sorry.

medical check-up. If there is a history of breast or cervical cancer, heart disease, high blood pressure, blood clotting problems or gall bladder disorders, a woman may be advised that the treatment is not suitable.

H.R.T. restores the balance of oestrogen and progesterone that the body has ceased to produce. Treatment can be prescribed in the form of a tablet or administered by sticking a patch which contains oestrogen on to the skin, in which case a progesterone pill would be taken in addition. Or a small pellet of oestrogen, the size of an apple pip, can be placed under the skin under local anaesthetic. Again, the progesterone would be taken by mouth.

Apart from the potential advantages I've already mentioned, H.R.T. can also help prevent osteoporosis or brittle bone disease. It can also help reduce the risk of heart disease.

However, some women may find that with the onset of regular periods again they might experience some breast tenderness and indeed medical opinion is divided on whether H.R.T. increases the risk of breast cancer.

Nevertheless, despite the controversy that surrounds it, I believe that women should be given the choice and H.R.T. should be made available to all those who might benefit from it and want to take advantage of another 25 years or so of quality life.

H.R.T. is just one of the advances in medical care that is now becoming more freely available to us. We women should also take advantage of the screening programmes that are now on offer. All women aged between 50 and 60 should be screened for breast cancer with a mammogram every three years. And all women, from the time they become sexually active, should take a smear test for cervical cancer every five years. It only takes two or three minutes and could save your life.

I can only emphasise how important these checks are from my own personal experience to prove to you that none of us is invincible.

Despite all the care I'd taken of my body, a routine mammogram revealed that I was in the early stages of breast cancer. Fortunately it had been detected at a stage where the diligence of the doctor who examined me paid off, and his referral to a cancer specialist allowed me to be treated successfully.

But I had cancer, and if I hadn't had that check-up then I would have had to face the inevitable. At first I couldn't believe it. But cancer is no respecter of age, class, or creed. Sometimes the only thing that can stop it in its tracks is early detection.

So please learn from my experience. Particularly if you are approaching middle age or the menopause, you should consider a complete all-round medical check-up – a bit like the M.O.T for a car. Just think of it as a testing out of your roadworthiness, a chance to correct some minor faults, and you'll enjoy smooth running for many years to come. It's also a time to check out your eyes and your teeth. If you catch a problem early, you'll avoid difficult times ahead. And don't be backward in coming forward to ask your doctor's advice on any other health problems. Knowledge and understanding of our health, and particularly women's health, has improved immeasurably over the past 30 or 40 years.

But whatever you do, remember that your continued good health depends on keeping up a well-balanced diet and plenty of exercise. Inactivity and ageing are not the same thing and neither is an excuse for the other. Keep at it and you'll keep your independence and stay young at heart.

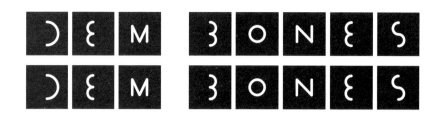

A few years ago I was enjoying skating on a local ice rink. A foolish slip put me out of action for six months with a very painful broken bone. The break at the wrist was typical, however, of those suffered by many middle-aged and elderly women through osteoporosis or brittle bone disease.

After intense physiotherapy and regular exercise I am happy to say that my arm recovered fully. But that break not only reinforced my belief in keeping fit and maintaining physical strength, especially as the years go by, it also fuelled an interest in osteoporosis.

The Amarant Centre in London is one of the country's leading clinics dealing with the menopause and H.R.T. Their work indicates that among its other many benefits, H.R.T. may lead to the strengthening of bones in menopausal women. Indeed, a primary cause of brittle bones is the drop in oestrogen and progesterone levels associated with the menopause. But a poor diet, smoking and excess alcohol, along with hereditary factors combined with inactivity, are also contributory factors.

Again, H.R.T. may not be the answer for you. You must take medical advice and feel free to go elsewhere for a second opinion. Remember, you must be in charge of what happens to your own body.

Nevertheless one in four women under 60 will sustain an osteoporotic fracture. And the figures go up to one in two by their 70s. Fractures occur most often in the wrist, hip and spine. And osteoporosis is not only a major cause of disability in the Western World, it can also prove fatal.

In some, bone decay can become so severe that it gradually affects the spine which painfully collapses, decreasing a woman's height by many inches and causing a curvature of the spine which is often referred to as a 'dowager's hump' – a cruel description for a painful condition which makes simple daily tasks like bending, stretching or lifting things up beyond a woman's capacity.

Throughout our childhood, the skeleton grows until at maturity it reaches its peak strength and fitness. At about 35 the bones of both men and women begin to lose their thickness and strength. But for women, the menopause can bring about a rapid decline.

Whether male or female, a lifetime of inactivity, smoking, drinking and poor nutrition only serves to make things much worse. Our bones are made of calcium, and benefit from a regular intake of fresh sources. You'll find it in milk (there's just as much in semi-skimmed), low-fat cheese, yogurt, bread, broccoli, sardines, baked beans and apricots. We can get all the Vitamin D we need from herrings, kippers, mackerel, sardines or a capsule of cod-liver oil. Vitamin D is also absorbed when we expose our bodies to sunlight. Not too much though, as recent studies into skin cancer tend to indicate.

But it's the menopause that makes the odds against women unfair and we should consider ourselves particularly at risk if our lives, particularly our working lives, have meant us sitting around hour in, hour out. Inactivity and bone disease are very closely linked. Even some of arguably the fittest men in the world – astronauts – experience dramatic loss of calcium in their bones after a short period of weightlessness.

For us earthbound mortal women H.R.T. can be the answer. But as I've said before, this treatment may not be suitable for all women.

But help is on the horizon in the shape of recent research which has proved that a healthy amount of exercise (like the exercises in this book) can prevent some bone loss and increase bone strength. The exercise must be weight-

TOP TIP

Alcohol is high in calories so check your intake. Women should not drink more than 14 units a week. There's one unit in a glass of wine or a half pint of lager. Drink sensibly and spread your units over the week, leaving some days alcohol free.

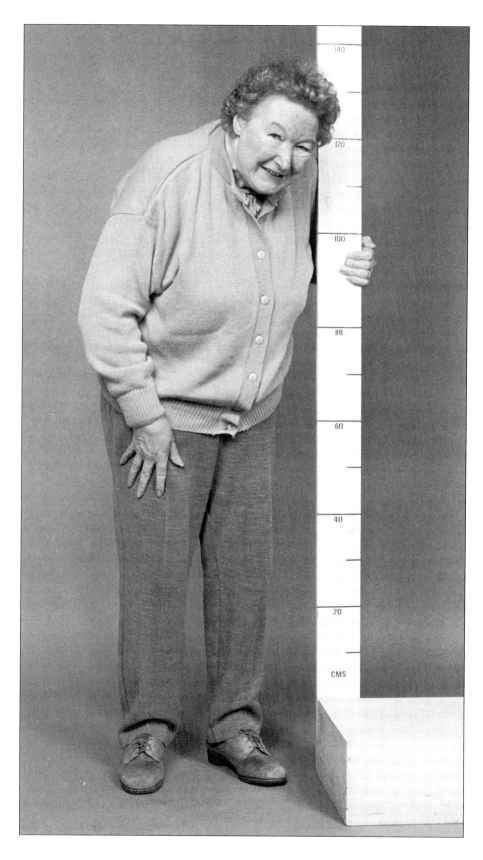

bearing, but that simply means making the most of the weight of your own body with brisk walking, jogging, exercising to music, or indeed anything that will strengthen the spine, hips and legs.

Our arms, too can benefit from weight-bearing exercises. And again, it's simple. Just lifting a can of beans up and down, carrying the shopping home, doing the gardening – they'll all help.

These weight-bearing exercises stress the bone and encourage fresh calcium deposits to strengthen it. But unfortunately osteoporosis cannot be reversed so it is essential to prevent it in the first place.

Remember this is a silent and insidious disease that makes women its first target. Those particularly at risk are women whose menopause came early or who have had a hysterectomy. So too are female athletes whose dedication to their sport disrupted their periods, and anorexics.

On the bright side, women who have had children or been on the contraceptive pill which contains oestrogen appear to be less at risks. As too are slightly plumper ladies, who seem to be less prone to osteoporosis than their smaller-framed friends.

Incidentally, a gentle ticking off for all those who have complained about the introduction of fluoride into our water supplies. Fluoride not only makes strong teeth, it also makes strong hearts and bones!

Lastly, if you already suffer from osteoporosis, you should not attempt the exercises in this book. And if you are in any doubt, you should consult your doctor first.

TOP TIP
Keep your body strong and you'll find that you'll be able to tackle everyday chores and problems a lot more easily. It really is true about a healthy body and a healthy mind!

Pictured opposite: The visual effect of osteoporosis with reference to curvature of the spine.

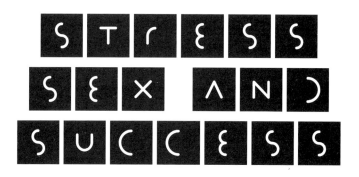

STRESS SEX AND SUCCESS

if, through following the advice in this book, you have **eased into fitness**, apart from feeling on top of the world you should also be much better equipped to deal with the bane of 20th century life – stress.

Our primitive ancestors knew next to nothing about stress. No problems with unpaid bills, traffic jams, sons and daughters who forgot to ring home!

All they had to cope with were the more immediate problems of marauding animals or aggressors. Their bodies simply geared up ready for a fight or, if discretion took the better part, a hasty flight.

Our bodies still react in the same way that our ancestors' did. The muscles tense, blood pressure increases the flow of adrenalin. We sweat, feel anger or anxiety, and start to breathe quickly. The liver releases sugar, cholesterol and fatty acids into the blood, and the body is ready for action.

Unfortunately we're not able to see the process through in the same way that our ancestors did. We don't actually fight or flee – not most of the time, anyway! In effect we've got the body all stressed up with nowhere to go and we're left with feelings of frustration, anxiety and over-stimulation. Constant stress like this cannot only lead to sleepless nights, it may also lead to physical and mental illness and muscular and digestive disorders. Many doctors believe, too, that some cancers are brought about by high stress levels.

But we have the remedy in our own hands. Our ancestors' response was physical, and so must ours be. Regular exercise, whether following the programme in this book or by walking, swimming or jogging, is the best antidote to stress and tension there is. Just remember to breathe properly, into your stomach and not just into your chest, and smooth those cares away.

Don' forget though that stress is very much part of our lives and we all need a certain amount. It's stress that pushes us on to achieve greater things and meet challenges. It's only when it becomes excessive that we risk illness.

Of course, there is another way to relieve stress and tension and, with love and affection, a far more pleasurable one – sexual intercourse. Indeed, one of the many benefits of a body that has been put in order with a healthy diet and regular exercise may well be an enhanced sex lie. You're looking good, you feel great, so why not?

Sex is great, but unsafe sex can kill. Many sexually transmitted diseases can be cured but the risk of infection and AIDS still remains. There is no vaccine to protect you against HIV infection and no cure for AIDS.

Do enjoy a healthy sex life. But bear in mind you can't tell whether a partner is infected just by looking at them. Please practise safe sex.

Remember, life is for living. If you've followed the words of advice in this book and learnt from my experiences, some good, some bad, then you can pat yourself on the back (you'll find it easier now!) and face the world and the future brimming with confidence.

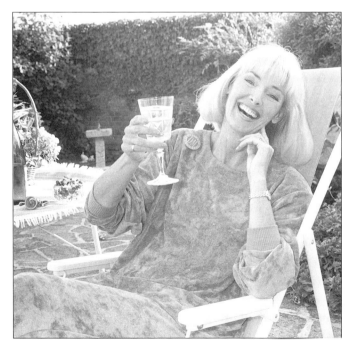

One last word of advice. Don't stop now. Keep at it. And keep on keeping fit!